THIS IS WHAT
YOU JUST PUT
IN YOUR MOUTH?

THIS IS WHAT YOU JUST PUT IN YOUR MOUTH?

From Eggnog to Beef Jerky, the Surprising Secrets
of What's Inside Everyday Products

Patrick Di Justo

THREE RIVERS PRESS • NEW YORK

All rights reserved.
Published in the United States by Three Rivers Press,
an imprint of the Crown Publishing Group,
a division of Random House LLC,
a Penguin Random House Company, New York.
www.crownpublishing.com

Three Rivers Press and the Tugboat design are registered
trademarks of Random House LLC.

Portions of this book have been adapted from material by the author that
first appeared in *Wired* magazine.

Library of Congress Cataloging-in-Publication Data
Di Justo, Patrick
This is what you just put in your mouth? : from eggnog to beef jerky, the
surprising secrets of what's inside everyday products / Patrick Di Justo.—
First edition.
pages cm
1. Food—Composition—Popular works.   2. Processed foods—Popular
works.   I. Title.
TX355.D54 2015
664'.07—dc23   2014043509

ISBN 978-0-8041-3988-5
eBook ISBN 978-0-8041-3989-2

Printed in the United States of America

Book design by Elizabeth Rendfleisch
Illustrations by Anders Wenngren
Cover design by Nupoor Gordon
Cover photography by Grounder/Shutterstock

10 9 8 7 6 5 4 3 2 1

First Edition

For Emily Gertz, who never stopped believing

Contents

Introduction

· ·

It started with a simple question. A bunch of us were sitting around at a Super Bowl party in the early 2000s. On the table in front of us was the usual array of snack foods that accompany a Super Bowl party: chicken wings, corn and potato chips, pretzels, pigs in blankets, hamantaschen ... the spread looked endless. Most of the stuff was easily identifiable, but there, in the middle of all the bowls of chips, was an orange-and-blue can of Kraft Easy Cheese. Spray-on cheese. Aerosol cheese in a can. A friend of mine, who shall remain a nameless drunk, picked up the can, stared at it like it was a totem pole, and asked, "Did you ever, like, really wonder what's, like, really in this?"

That simple intoxicated query started me on the eight-year quest that has led to the book you're holding in your hands. At the time I was writing for *Wired* magazine, and I pitched the idea to my editor Laura Moorhead: what if we devoted a page of the magazine every month to really looking into the ingredients of everyday household products? I could interview scientists and doctors and inventors and food manufacturers and product marketers—everyone would want to talk about their products!

Two years later, they accepted my pitch, and the first article ran in the October 2006 issue. After that, I had a product investigation in nearly every issue until October 2013.

My hope is that these columns harken back to the old days of journalism, when reporters had the time and backing to really do investigative reporting. To get to the bottom of some of these products, I've interviewed dozens of people, exchanged e-mails with hundreds more, visited shiny new laboratories and dusty deserted libraries. Once, I even broke Google. I learned more than I ever thought I could about chemistry and biology, about material science, about the laws concerning food and drugs and advertising, and about the immaterial ways of human nature. I found people who were extraordinarily generous with their time and their knowledge—when's the last time you explained your job in detail to a total stranger who called and asked?—and I found people who really, really, really seemed not to like, or even to understand, the idea of a free press.

Generally, creating these columns worked like this: I'd query friends, family, colleagues, and strangers on the Internet. They would suggest products to investigate, sometimes because they really wanted to know, sometimes because they just wanted to be scared of what I would find. I also got a lot of product ideas simply by taking a shopping cart up and down the aisles of my local supermarket or big-box store.

At some point very early in the month, I'd put together a list of products I wanted to investigate and clear it with my editor. He or she would make some suggestions, and then I'd get to work.

The investigation usually started with a phone call or e-mail to the product's parent company. Most companies that create products found on supermarket shelves are gigantic conglomerates, and they typically have a well-staffed media center that handles questions from reporters without troubling executive management. The PR departments of Kraft, Nestlé, and Procter & Gamble were definitely on my speed dial. But there are some very famous products, like cherry cordials and Samuel Adams beer, that are made by companies one step up from mom-and-pop operations, where many of the employees are the family of the founders. For those companies, a call to the main office will more than likely be answered by someone who can directly talk with the president of the company.

I started each call by explaining my mission. I was writing an article about their fine product. I would be looking at every single ingredient: what it does, how it fits into the product, and how it works with other ingredients to make the product do what it does. I would be also talking to doctors and professors, really to anyone who could help explain the ingredients of this product.

In these conversations, I always made it clear that I was starting with the company, to give them the fullest chance to be a part of my research into this product. More often than not, the people I spoke to were thrilled to hear from me. More than anything, a manufacturer wants publicity for their product. And there is nothing like having a full, glossy magazine page devoted entirely to your product to get that kind of publicity. Small companies would usually willingly set up a time for a telephone interview with their president. Employees of a large corporation would always have to check with someone, but they usually did this with great glee; it's not every day that the publicity of having your product in a major magazine falls into your lap.

Unfortunately, this was also the moment when trouble began. The people I spoke to would get off the phone and Google my name, looking up previous examples of my work to see exactly how these stories turned out. I was never there in the room when they did this, but I dreaded to think of their hopeful faces crashing in sheer horror. "What have I gotten my product into?" they must have wondered. The articles they saw didn't sing the praises of the products, accompanied by beautiful pictures that showed the objects in the best light. No, these poor people were looking at investigative, sometimes even sarcastic, stories that didn't pull any punches. One cardinal rule of corporate public relations: you almost never want to tell it as it is.

While this was happening I would be tearing up the Google machine and the interlibrary loan network to get as much information as I could about this product's various ingredients. The important thing when using Google was never to stop at the first page; Google page results really don't get interesting until you go about ten or even twenty screens deep.

By the next day or the day after, I'd hear back from the person I spoke to (if they really were in shock, I'd have to reach out to them). Many times their prior enthusiasm was replaced by a dull depression, in which even feeling bad was too much of an effort. Sometimes they would say that upon reflection they didn't think their product was a good fit for the story I wanted to do. Sometimes they would say straight out that they wanted absolutely nothing to do with a magazine column that seriously looked into the ingredients of their products. Sometimes they thought that would make me stop.

The rest of the month would be spent continuing to investigate ingredients, talking to scientists, talking to government officials, talking to professors, sometimes even talking to lawyers, to find out exactly what goes into the things we use in our everyday lives. There would almost always be some late nights, and some last-minute phone calls and e-mails, but I'd always have a finished story ready for my first-of-the-month deadline.

One quick word before we begin: If you're looking for shocking stories of the gigantic corporate conspiracy to poison America through its processed foods, you're reading the wrong book. This book's purpose isn't to scare you, or to enrage you, or to get you to e-mail your congressman. I never wrote any of these stories to "take down" any product. I always approached each product with nothing but curiosity and a desire to have that curiosity satisfied. It may not be the most important philosophical question in human existence to wonder what is inside a Slim Jim meat stick. But Slim Jims (along with Cool Whip, and Red Bull, and Head & Shoulders shampoo, and all the other products in this book) are a part of our world, and even if you don't use them, you are better off knowing what is in them rather than not knowing.

. . . .

PART ONE

THIS IS WHAT YOU
PUT IN YOUR MOUTH

This Is What You Put on Your Meat

A.1. Steak Sauce

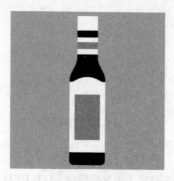

*A sauce of sulfur-based compounds, a saliva prompter,
and thick gooey bacterial excretions.*

NOTE: For this story I was privileged to interview noted chef Alton Brown, who was generous enough to share with me some of his thoughts on the ingredients.

Tomatoes

Pureed berries from the famously toxic nightshade family. The leaves and stems are poisonous, but the fruit is eminently edible. All tomatoes—not just varieties called "beefsteak"—contain about 0.25 percent glutamic acid, one of the savory chemicals that give beef its meatiness. Concentrated tomato fiber also imparts thickness.

> **Alton Brown:** *Tomatoes, like mushrooms, aged cheeses, red wine, and beef, contain amino acids that deliver meaty flavors that have become known as "umami." Adding them to a steak can help to turn the flavor up to eleven.*

Raisin Paste

A key ingredient since chef H. W. Brand added it to King George IV's steak sauce in the 1820s. Raisins contain antioxidants, which may have helped mask the rancid flavor of spoiling meat in the days before refrigeration.

Alton Brown: *The inclusion of raisin paste is genius. The ultimate accompaniment to a steak is a glass of red wine, again due to the complex "umami" effect. Wine is made from grapes, raisins are grapes, so it's a natural. Raisin paste also serves as a binder and in this case a replacement for fats such as olive oil.*

Distilled Vinegar

One of the oldest meat tenderizers. Earlier versions of A.1. used tastier (but more expensive) malt vinegar, which is made from unhopped beer. The distilled variety is made from industrial vats of pure ethanol, fermented by rod-shaped *Acetobacter* bacteria.

Alton Brown: *Vinegar contains acetic acid, and in the mouth acids prompt the release of the ultimate meat tenderizer: saliva. Acidity also helps to balance sweetness and enhance aromatic qualities. Once upon a time A.1. was formulated with malt vinegar, which is full of complex flavors created during the malting process of barley. These days they use cheap distilled vinegar. So much for complexity.*

Corn Syrup

Here, as in so many other American foods, corn syrup is used as a sweetener and thickener. Early advertisements described this stuff as "pre-digested" and ready for use by the blood, like that's a good thing. Well, during World War II, it was a good thing: donated red blood cells were concentrated and stored in corn syrup before use.

Alton Brown: *A small amount of sweetness does enhance the flavors created by a good sear, but the tomato paste in A.1. covers that base just fine. The corn syrup here functions as a texture adjuster, smoothing out any grit from the tomato puree. It gives the sauce "cling" to hold on to the target food. It masks "off" flavors (ask Mary Poppins about that one) and it gives Americans what they like best of all: sweetness.*

Salt

Salt, sugar, and meaty umami flavor are positive tastes, leading us toward nutrients; bitter and sour are negative, driving us away from alkalines and acids. When salt hits the taste buds, it suppresses the perception of bitterness. One tablespoon of A.1. (and, really, who uses that little?) contains an eighth of your recommended daily dosage of sodium.

Alton Brown: The word "sauce" ultimately derives from the Latin "sal," meaning "salt," so this is the only ingredient that makes absolute sense. Besides the fact that salt just plain tastes good, some say it has a very special effect on taste buds, essentially amplifying their detection abilities. Above all, salt counteracts sweetness. Without it, A.1. would be a dessert sauce.

Crushed Orange Puree

Older versions of A.1. used marmalade made with bittersweet Seville oranges. The switch to a puree is likely more apparent to the nose than to the tongue.

Alton Brown: The very unique bitterness of marmalade combined with the gamey acidity of the malt vinegar made for a pretty great sauce. Replacing the pricier marmalade with crushed orange puree grants A.1. a bit of complexity, but most of the citrus is detected in the nose rather than the mouth. It also helps to cover the jaggedness of the distilled vinegar.

Dried Garlic and Onion

Beef has scores of sulfur-based flavor compounds, most notably hydrogen sulfide. Since garlic and onions also contain sulfur compounds, they can help make even the lousiest cuts taste richer and "meatier."

Alton Brown: This is one case where the dried version is superior to fresh. Not only are dried garlic and onion more powerful

than raw forms, since they're standardized products their
performance is predictable.

. . . .

Spices and Herbs

A corporate secret, of course.

*Alton Brown: Legally, a food manufacturer does not have to
list herbs and spices by name. I can't detect any individual
spice flavors in A.1. but if I were to make my own I'd reach for
dry mushroom powder, allspice, white pepper, and anchovy (not
technically a spice but a powerful flavorant nonetheless).*

. . . .

Caramel Color

Sugar or similar carbohydrates browned at about 130 degrees
Fahrenheit. The brown tint eliminates the red of the tomatoes.

*Alton Brown: Humans eat with their eyes first and caramel color
says "sear," which is what we want on a steak. Without it, A.1.
would look like spaghetti sauce, or worse yet . . . ketchup.*

. . . .

Xanthan Gum

A polysaccharide excreted by the *Xanthomonas campestris*
bacterium, this gummy substance has a peculiar viscosity: it
thickens the mix, stabilizing the ingredients, but when shaken or
poured, it behaves in a more liquid manner.

. . . .

[BACKSTORY]

I love A.1. I can practically eat it with a spoon.

We came up with the idea of interviewing the great chefs of television to get their opinions and insights into A.1. I contacted the representatives for Rachael Ray, Wolfgang Puck, Paula Deen, Alain Ducasse, Mario Batali, Nigella Lawson, Emeril Lagasse, Alice Waters, Anthony Bourdain, Jamie Oliver, and Tom Colicchio. None of them were willing or able to help. Most of them didn't even respond. Bobby Flay's people said he would, but then Flay flaked.

Only Alton Brown came through, and boy did he ever come through! He gave intelligent, well-thought-out answers to our questions and offered his insights into what the secret herbs and spices might be. I can't say enough good things about Alton Brown.

The research for these stories doesn't stop with just the current ingredient list. As conglomerates buy up small mom-and-pop companies, they tend to subtly change the

---

NATURAL FLAVORINGS, ARTIFICIAL FLAVORINGS, SPICES
Natural flavorings are the oil, essence, extract, or distillates that contain the flavor chemicals from spices; fruits; vegetables; herbs; bark, roots, leaves, or similar plant material; meat; poultry; seafood; or dairy products, which are primarily used as flavorings and not for nutrition.

Artificial flavorings are any substance (and that's the exact phrase in the FDA document: "any substance") that is used to impart flavor to a product and does not meet the definition of a natural flavoring.

Spices are aromatic vegetable substances whose significant function in food is seasoning rather than nutrition.

formulation of their newly acquired products, either to make them cheaper to produce or to better fit into the company's manufacturing flow. I had a sneaking suspicion that A.1., which had been passed around several companies since the 1980s, was extremely likely to have been reformulated over the years.

But how do you find out the ingredients that *were* in a product thirty or sixty years ago? Especially if the new parent company doesn't want to help you (and might not even know the pre-buyout formulation)? You do what I did: turn to our old friend the Internet.

Find the November 5, 1956, issue of *Life* magazine in Google Books. Preview the issue, and scroll down to page 79. You'll see a full-page, full-color broiled steak, with a bottle of A.1. steak sauce standing before it like a conqueror. Now zoom in on the label. Google scanned these magazines at such high resolution that you can clearly read the ingredient list on the bottle and can compare it to the current ingredient list. Kids, this is how you get information that no one else seems to have.

While you have that image in front of you, look at the next-to-last item in the ingredient list. A.1. used to contain a substance called "tragacanth." It's not in the modern variety at all. A little research found that tragacanth is a tree sap, commonly used back then as a thickener (probably before the development of xanthan gum). It's used in very few foods today. I wonder what tragacanth tasted like.

This Is What You Put in Your Dog

Purina Alpo Chop House Beef Tenderloin Flavor in Gourmet Gravy

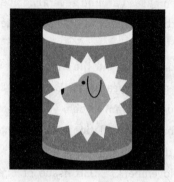

Chicken, corn, wheat, and an unknown liver, flavored to taste like beef.

Poultry

Here's the dirty little secret. Poultry, according to the FDA, can be *any domesticated bird*: chickens, turkeys, ducks, and geese. But it can also include creatures that you don't find in as many storybooks, like ostriches, emus, squabs, guinea hens, pheasants, partridges, quails, or pigeons. Fido probably wouldn't have a problem eating any of those birds, but knowing the public outcry that would happen if Alpo were made of pigeons, it's probably a safe bet that this ingredient is either chicken or turkey, according to availability (i.e., whichever bird happens to be cheaper in the commodities market on the day the Alpo factory buys its raw materials).

Liver

Rich in iron, liver is your pet's "hot button"—when dogs kill in the wild, they will usually devour the liver and other organs first. The problem is that Alpo is not a wild kill; it comes from an animal-processing plant, and the ingredient list never specifies exactly *whose* liver it is. We're pretty sure it's not horse. While horsemeat used to be a staple of dog food, at the time of this writing the last horse abattoir in the US closed in 2007.

Wheat Gluten
The rubbery high-protein concentrate that's left over after a wheat kernel has had its carbohydrates removed. (The flavored variety in your local Whole Foods is commonly called seitan, and it is used as a meat substitute in vegetarian diets.) It's made of two proteins: gliadin, which is the sticky toxin responsible for celiac disease, and glutenin, which shares the same Latin root as *gluten* and *glue*. This gives dough its strength and elasticity. Something like 0.75 percent (three-quarters of 1 percent) of healthy American humans are sensitive to gliadin (the stat always seems to be mentioned in relation to "healthy" people) but dogs may be different; in a 1937 study, six dogs fed high-gliadin diets (in the range of 16–25 percent of total caloric intake) all had reactions that bore a striking resemblance to epileptic convulsions, most likely due to becoming sensitized to the protein. Also, dogs fed high-gliadin diets developed a deficiency in the vital amino acid lysine.

Soy Flour
Ground-up soybeans, rich in lysine. Wouldn't you know. For a product with the word "beef" in the title, we have to wonder just how much of these vegetable-derived proteins are in Alpo. In fact, the FDA warns consumers about this possibility when choosing a pet food: even though poultry is the first ingredient, the wheat and soy products—when added together—may turn out to be the most abundant protein in this product.

Meat By-products
Societies that eat animals usually are in agreement about eating animal muscle; few omnivores dislike sirloin, chicken breast, or ham hocks. But different cultures have differing views of eating

animal organs or entrails. Affluent white Anglozone Americans often shun things like hearts and lungs, while other cultures treat those and other organs like delicacies. Modern life is all about efficiency, using every last bit of what we have, so meat processors usually have no problem selling lungs, spleens, kidneys, brains, blood, bones, some fatty tissue, and stomach and intestines as dog food. It may sound pretty disgusting to us, but remember, thirty thousand years ago, your precious little Fido was still a wolf. If he reverted and began hunting livestock on his own, there's no way he would leave those juicy bits behind.

Beef

Finally! Beef! The legal definition of beef stretches like a pair of Spanx to include striated skeletal muscle, tongue, diaphragm, heart, esophagus, and overlying fat, and the skin, sinew, nerves, and blood vessels normally found with that flesh. But wait: doesn't the label say that this must be "beef tenderloin"? Not at all. The label calls for "beef tenderloin *flavor.*" Based on its appearance underneath meat by-products on the label, there just might be more spleen than sirloin in Alpo.

Modified Cornstarch

Regular cornstarch turns into a thick, cloudy gel with the addition of liquids and heat. Modified cornstarch, when wetted and heated, becomes a clear mucuslike gel, excellent for filling fruit pies. What's the difference? Instead of stretching out in a chain, modified cornstarch molecules are cross-linked to one another. That way, they swell with water just like regular starch but don't break down and become opaque. The FDA-approved chemicals for modifying cornstarch include hydrochloric and sulfuric acids, hydrogen peroxide, chlorine, and sodium chloride.

Calcium Phosphate

Bones. But not really. Vertebrate bones (is "vertebrate bones" redundant?), which dogs love to crunch on, are made of a specific type of calcium phosphate known as hydroxyapatite. But there's a specific FDA category for "bone meal," which is used on ingredient lists when real bones are employed in domestic animal feed. So what is this stuff? It is very much like bones without actually being bones. It is the mineral form of calcium phosphate, which can be dug out of the ground and added to Alpo to provide necessary calcium for your canine. The good news is that you need less of this stuff to match the equivalent of bone meal, plus you avoid any risk of bovine spongiform encephalopathy (a.k.a. "mad cow") disease being passed along. (This is a good thing; dogs don't appear to be susceptible to the disease, but why risk it?) The bad news is that too much mined calcium phosphate can lead to calcium uroliths (a.k.a. doggie bladder stones), particularly in the little yappy breeds like Yorkshire terriers.

Natural Flavor

According to the FDA, pet foods often contain "digests," which are materials treated with heat, enzymes, and/or acids to form concentrated natural flavors. But what flavor? Liver? Poultry? Beef? Death? Your dog, being part scavenger, is naturally drawn to the smell of relatively newly dead carrion; pet food manufacturers know this and do what they can to make their wet food deliberately stinky. But not too stinky; a really bad-smelling pet food might entice a dog but can be too repulsive for the humans who have to shell out money to buy the stuff.

[BACKSTORY]

The trouble started when I asked Alpo, "Whose liver is this?"

As I explained earlier, when I research a product, I first contact the company. They're all excited to hear that someone wants to write about their product. Then I ask some questions, and they often clam up and never want to hear from me again.

That's what happened here. The folks at Alpo, a subsidiary of Purina, itself a subsidiary of Nestlé, were thrilled at first when I wanted to write about Alpo Chop House Beef Tenderloin Flavor in Gourmet Gravy. Most corporate communications people are trained to believe that every bit of publicity helps. But when I started asking about meat by-products and liver, they reverted to corporatespeak:

> Patrick, thanks for touching base again. We'd just like to reiterate that ALPO® is a premium quality product; that all ALPO® products are 100 percent complete and balanced for dogs, and that all ingredients are listed on the package in compliance with pet food regulatory standards. We appreciate the loyalty and trust of the millions of dog lovers who have fed and continue to feed ALPO® to their dogs. Thank you again for your interest in our products.

I always take statements like this to mean, "Go away! We're not breaking the law!" Which is a far cry from telling us whose liver this is. Of course, I didn't go away. I was frankly amazed that pet food manufacturers don't have to say where they get their liver.

Why the focus on liver? Because the liver is the body's

FRESH, FROZEN, AND THE POLITICS OF "HARD CHILLED"

In the mid-1990s, the United States Department of Agriculture decided to do something about frozen chicken. Specifically, they wanted to start calling it "frozen chicken." Up till then, a chicken that was frozen as solid as a block of ice could still technically be labeled "fresh" chicken. After lengthy hearings, in August 1995 the USDA redefined "fresh" to mean poultry whose internal temperature has never been below twenty-six degrees Fahrenheit (the temperature at which raw chicken freezes solid). Chicken that had been stored between twenty-six degrees Fahrenheit and zero degrees Fahrenheit would now receive a new label: "hard chilled." The ruling was published in the *Federal Register* in January 1996 and got instant media attention. The *New York Times* in particular was effusive that sanity now reigned in the USDA and that chicken frozen solid would no longer get to be called fresh.

But remember, this was 1995, and Congress was Newt Gingrich's Contract with America Congress, the first Republican Congress in forty-two years, and they wanted nothing to do with increased federal regulation of any business. So Congress deliberately refused to appropriate money to allow the USDA to enforce the hard-chilled rule. (And as we'll see in later chapters, if a food ruling isn't going to be enforced, some manufacturers can act as if it doesn't even exist.) Congress instead requested that the USDA "rethink" the definition of "fresh."

The folks at the USDA got the hint. Almost immediately, the old new rule was rescinded and a new new rule took its place. Now chicken that has been stored below twenty-six degrees Fahrenheit can no longer be called fresh, but neither does it have to be called hard chilled. At least chicken stored below zero degrees Fahrenheit would still be called frozen. The new law took effect December 17, 1997.

great filter. It removes a number of different toxins from the bloodstream, and as with the air filter on a car or the dust filter in an air conditioner, those toxins *can* accumulate in the liver before they are expelled and/or processed. The FDA lists no fewer than twenty-nine different substances, from antibiotics to pesticides, that can accumulate in animal liver. Shouldn't we know where that liver's been?

But I suspect that this ties into the bizarre reality about pet food in America: pet foods are formulated for the human owners of pets, maybe more so than for the pets themselves.

For example, in their advertisements in *Life* magazine in the 1950s, Ken-L Ration dog food bragged that it was made with "lean, red US Government inspected horsemeat." Nowadays, even if horsemeat were competitive on a price basis with other meats (and it's hard to imagine an economy where it's cheaper to truck in horsemeat from Mexico instead of chicken livers from a local farm), I strongly doubt you'd ever see *horse* on a label of dog food, even though your dog might relish the smelly, gamey quality of horsemeat. Why?

Because pet food manufacturers know there's a good chance that you, the human who buys food for your dog, will be turned off by horsemeat. It's the same thinking that makes pet food makers brag about the vegetables in their cat food, even though your cat, as an obligate carnivore, doesn't need vegetables: *you* feel that your cat should have a "balanced" diet of meat and veggies, so the pet food makers adjust the formula to give you what you want (and possibly to lower their own costs), even if your cat couldn't care less. And so it really doesn't matter how much your dog wants it; you're not likely to feed My Little Pony to your big Great Dane.

Based on my analysis of prices, laws, and the rather nebulous phrase *regulatory standards*, I'm convinced that the liver in Alpo is either beef, poultry, pork, or lamb, or a mixture of all of them, purchased according to whatever is available most cheaply on the commodities markets that day. If the folks at Nestlé/Purina/Alpo simply admitted that, I wouldn't have thought twice about the provenance of Alpo's liver. It's when they don't come out and say where they get their liver that people start questioning; the whole "I don't have to tell you where I got my liver" attitude they get when they're asked . . . well, it can't help but make people suspicious. And the only thing they're hiding is the awkward likelihood that on any given day, they honestly don't know whose liver is in Alpo.

This Is What You Eat with Your Burrito

Beano

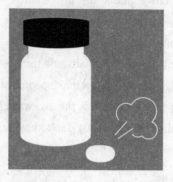

A dusty black enzyme that fixes a human genetic failing.

Alpha-Galactosidase

This enzyme does the work your small intestine won't. Beans (along with broccoli, cauliflower, and Brussels sprouts—all the musical fruits) contain complex carbs like raffinose that single-stomached animals like pigs, chickens, and humans are unable to digest. These carbs pass into the lower intestine intact, where bacteria turn them into CO_2, hydrogen, methane, and sulfur compounds that must find release. Alpha-galactosidase extracted from *Aspergillus niger* (the dusty black mold on old onions), with the help of a little bit of water, can break up raffinose, leaving behind simpler galactose and sucrose molecules for easier digestion and less putrefaction.

Invertase

Another enzyme, which further breaks the sucrose down into glucose and fructose—less wind-prone sugars. That said, Beano may cause a problem for people with diabetes, who weren't expecting cabbages to be broken down into the sugars sucrose, glucose, or fructose, none of which they need in their lives. The dilemma is whether to fart more or absorb about four extra grams of carbs for every one hundred grams of Beano-doped food they eat.

Cellulose Gel

As with most pills, the active ingredients in Beano (the alpha-galac enzymes) make up only a small part of the volume; the rest are what the industry calls excipients—inert ingredients that help deliver the dose. This microcrystalline cellulose (90 percent derived from wood pulp, 10 percent derived from the cell walls of cotton plants) acts as a filler, which is vital to pharmaceutical tablet-making: it binds everything together, then breaks apart easily in the gut.

Potato Starch

Like the Kardashians, industrial-quality potato starch is a flavorless, odorless, colorless substance that exists mainly to take up space. Here it also serves as a disintegrant: by absorbing water in the stomach, it causes the tablet to disintegrate, thus releasing the alpha-galac to do its enzymatic voodoo.

Colloidal Silica

These are nanoparticles that are chemically similar to unbelievably tiny particles of crushed beach sand. The pharma world calls this a glidant—an ultrafine powder that coats the other ingredients before they're poured into the mold, allowing them to flow past one another during the manufacturing process.

Magnesium Stearate

The "scum" in soap scum, here put to good use. Pill makers add this powdered lubricant to the mix to keep other powdered ingredients from gumming up their machines. But it takes only a tad, about 0.5 percent of the total pill; too much of this slippery stuff would prevent the tablet from holding together in the first place.

. . . .

Mannitol

A mildly sweet sugar alcohol with a nice mouthfeel that makes the medicine go down in a most delightful way. Curiously, high doses of sugar alcohols (like you might get from chewing too many sticks of sugar-free gum) can cause intestinal distress, including bloating, diarrhea, and . . . explosive flatulence.

. . . .

Sometimes corporate PR people are mother lodes of good, useful information (see the chapter on Tide Pods). Sometimes they're merely slightly helpful; sometimes they're not helpful at all. And sometimes they inadvertently give you the runaround.

Nearly every industry in the United States has a trade association. The American Dairy Council works on behalf of dairy farmers, the National Corn Growers Association works for corn growers, the United States Telecom Association stands with the US telecommunications industry, and even the Independent Community Bankers of America supports the independent community bankers. These trade associations are usually headquartered in Washington, DC, and many people think of them as nothing but lobbyists. The term "lobbyist" arose from a stereotype of their behavior: these were the people who waited around the lobby of the House and Senate for a moment when they could buttonhole a passing legislator and tell him all about their wonderful industry and what simple, harmless favors that senator or congressman could do for that industry. In return, the industry could

ENZYMES

Some chemical reactions, particularly the ones involved in keeping living things living, can be very hard to activate. They may require very high temperatures, or high concentrations of acid, or some other kind of life-threatening condition to get started. Enzymes are proteins that act as a special kind of catalyst—a substance that can lower the activation threshold for specific chemical reactions—allowing the process of life to take place at a more normal temperature or environment.

promise that politician their support: sometimes money in the form of campaign contributions (which are sometimes bribes in everything but the legal sense) and sometimes votes from their unified membership. It's even led to the coining of the ridiculous verb "to lobby," which is to advocate for a cause behind the scenes.

Reporters need to deal with these various trade associations, because the people in these associations know a great deal about the industry and can answer most questions. If they can't, their knowledge of everyone-who-is-anyone in their field can quickly get you to the right phone; if you want to find the one person in America who knows the most about cement drying times, you go to the National Council For Cement and Building Materials: they'll know exactly whom you should talk to.

Usually.

As I was writing this story, I got the idea to check one last thing—I wanted to know exactly what modified potato starch was and what chemicals were used to modify it. It was kind of last-minute, but some of the greatest parts of stories have arisen from a last-minute question.

I called the Potato Association of America ("A Professional Society for Advancement of the Potato Industry") to ask a simple question: "What is modified potato starch, and how is it modified?" Their PR person said, "Wow, we love questions like that from the media. I'm going to pass you on to the National Potato Council, because they have the experts who can answer that sort of thing."

The PR person for the National Potato Council ("Standing Up for Potatoes on Capitol Hill") said, "Hmmmmm, we're just a lobbying firm. You'd want to talk to someone at our scientific sister organization, the US Potato Board."

The PR person for the US Potato Board ("Maximizing Return on Grower Investment") said, "Wow, such an exciting question. You know who's the real experts on this? The people at National Starch. I'm going to pass you on to them; their number is . . ."

"Good morning, National Starch—unleashing the power of starchology, how may I direct your call?" I told them I had a simple question: "What is modified potato starch, and what are the physical/chemical processes by which it is modified?" The PR person who took the call said she knew just the person in their organization who could help me, especially since I'd been bounced around so much. She connected me with his voice mail.

The guy was on vacation until February 13, long after the story's deadline, so we never had the chance to find out how potato starch is modified. This happens every so often: sometimes you really nail the story; sometimes the story really nails you.

This Is What You Put in Your Mouth

Chocolate Cherry Cordials

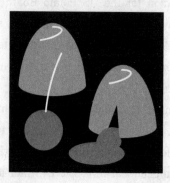

It's not spit. It's not. But it's kind of like spit.

Maraschino Cherry

The heart of this candy, and the heart of this candy's conundrum: how exactly do they get the liquid center outside the cherry yet *inside* the chocolate shell? Historically, these were Balkan cherries infused with a delicate Marasca liqueur, but that was then; these modern maraschinos mostly come from Michigan and are a little less cultured: their infusion is corn syrup and high-fructose corn syrup.

Red Dye #40

A maraschino's unnaturally red color is, in fact, unnatural: Red Dye #40 is a nitrogen-based (a.k.a. "azo") dye derived from petroleum. Some Euro nations require labeling saying that 40 can have a negative impact on children; in the US, the Center for Science in the Public Interest says that 40's key safety studies were flawed. They want the FDA to ban the dye; the FDA is thinking about it.

Sulfur Dioxide

This simple chemical is added to some fruits to block the oxygen-enzyme reaction that can turn fruit brown. Generally safe for most humans, SO_2 can trigger an asthma attack (close to anaphylactic shock!) in susceptible individuals. One odd note: this chemical destroys the vitamin B1 molecule, a harsh wakeup for those who thought maraschino cherries were a health food.

Sugar

A sucrose solution is heated to a 185 degree slurry and poured into a mold. The cherry is added, then more sugar solution; the final cooled result is a white "bullet" of solid sugar with a cherry inside.

Invertase

Does digestion begin in the mouth or in the factory? This digestive enzyme is commonly found in human saliva and in the small intestine (though confectionery invertase comes from yeast, if that makes you feel any better). It is added to the still-warm sugar, where it immediately starts, well, *digesting* the sucrose into its constituent glucose and fructose.

Milk Chocolate Coating

Applied to the sugar-cherry bullet in a kind of Willy Wonka waterfall, this seals in the cherry, sugar, and invertase. Over the course of the next few weeks, the enzyme uses the water in the cherry to break down—the manufacturers use the word "hydrolyze"—the sucrose molecules into the magical liquid center everyone expects.

PGPR

The public name for polyglycerol polyricinoleate, a relatively new addition to the FDA's allowed food additives. This stuff is an emulsifier, laboratory-made out of glycerol and ricinoleic acids from castor beans. Why do some of the biggest names in chocolate go through the trouble of adding this to their chocolate, when natural cocoa butter does the same job and comes with the bean? Almost all chocolate that goes through production equipment will use one of two approved emulsifiers for chocolate, soya lecithin or PGPR. Presently PGPR is less expensive.

. . . .

Vanillin

If you can create this exact molecule—responsible for the odor and taste of vanilla—using chemicals in a laboratory, is it the same as "real" vanilla? This question could keep the Philosophy 101 students up all night, but the US government is more pragmatic: it says only vanillin from vanilla beans is natural. Anyway, it's a moot point: almost 87 percent of all vanillin in the world is the synthetic kind.

. . . .

MARASCHINO CHERRIES

Consider the lowly pickle, a preserved cucumber that still has a slightly crunchy consistency if made properly. Like a pickle, cordial manufacturers want to preserve the character of the cherry in making a maraschino. They don't want it to be mushy or flat like canned cherries or frozen cherries after thawing. So at harvest they immerse the cherry in a briny solution of salt and SO_2 to arrest the enzymatic function that breaks down the sugars, causing decay in fruit. The SO_2 also prevents browning (which is why it is commonly found in things like white wine, fresh sliced apples in a salad bar, lettuce, etc.), because the browning is the result of the decaying process arrested in the brining. There is also a slight bleaching effect on the cherries as any light red pigment in the skin is broken down and dissolved, leaving a "pickled" yellow cherry.

If the brine is maintained at the proper level of salt and SO_2, the cherries will remain in a neutral stable state for many months. When manufacturers are ready to remove the pits and make maraschinos, they wash the cherries thoroughly to remove the salts and lower the SO_2 to a level well below fifty parts per million. They slowly add color (Red Dye #40) and sugar solids to the specified formulation. Cherry flavor is added at the end of the process in cover syrup. In essence, they remove the "cherryness" from the cherry, then put it back in months later.

[BACKSTORY]

I want to make this absolutely clear: there is no human saliva in cherry cordials. There are no nozzles spraying drool on the cherry; no one has the job of spitting on the candy as it goes by on a conveyer belt. No saliva in cherry cordials. None.

There are, however, artificial human salivary enzymes in cherry cordials.

Digestion starts in the mouth, with saliva enzymes. It continues through the stomach and into the small intestine, where other enzymes also contribute to digestion. Since invertase is found both in the mouth and in the small intestine, it is part of the digestive process. When invertase is sprayed on the sugar-coated cherry, the enzymatic breakdown starts within twenty-four hours. Within three weeks, the sugar coating has been completely liquefied, or "cordialized."

In other words—and there's no way around it—cherry cordials are predigested for you.

This Is What You Put Between Your Lips

Cigarettes

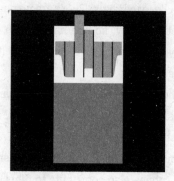

Cheesy foot smell, beaver juice, and the original smokable weed.

Tobacco

Thanks to nicotine—a plant alkaloid originally evolved by the plant world to be an antiherbivore—this weed may be mildly hallucinogenic. It can be chewed, brewed, smoked, or, as some South American shamans prefer, enjoyed as an enema.

Paper

Tobacco firms are very secretive about their products' myriad ingredients, but we do know that about 10 percent of any given smoke is simply the paper wrapping—cellulose and a thin strip of adhesive.

Menthol

The only additive the tobacco companies actually talk about, menthol is a mint derivative that causes local anesthesia and bronchodilation. This allows users to bring the smoke more deeply into the lungs, where nicotine and other combustion products can be more efficiently absorbed.

Ammonium Hydroxide

Essentially ammonia in water. There is some evidence that ammonia reacts with tobacco to free the nicotine, making it more accessible to the bloodstream (manufacturers dispute this). Of course, the material safety data sheet for this substance warns that inhaling ammonia vapors, whatever the source, may damage the upper respiratory tract.

Castoreum

Commonly found in the secretions of a beaver's castor glands (located near the animal's genitals), this substance when processed gives your cigarette a sweet odor and smoky flavor. In 1991, Philip Morris used just eight pounds of the pungent stuff to make four hundred billion cigarettes—proving that a little genital secretion goes a long way.

2-Acetyl-3-Ethylpyrazine

According to tobacco-industry documents, this pyrazine (an aromatic ringed compound) provides an "earthy depth of flavor." Funny, when the same compound is used in food preparation, it's described as tasting like potatoes.

Copaiba Oil

One way that Brazil intends to make itself independent of fossil fuels is with the oleoresin of the copaiba tree, which is so flammable it can practically fuel a diesel engine without any refining at all. Why is it in cigarettes? One possibility is that ammonium hydroxide decreases combustibility, so manufacturers have to counteract it with a nontoxic accelerant. Perhaps, but copaiba oil is also used as a folk remedy for prostate tumors (and gonorrhea). We're putting our money on the accelerant theory.

Phenyl Methyl Ketone (Acetophenone)

$C_6H_5COCH_3$ is a major component of tear gas, which should come as no surprise to anyone who's ever dealt with a cigarette left smoldering in an ashtray. Here it may act as a low-level narcotic.

Gamma-Heptalactone

This compound is a mild inhibitor of the CYP_2A_6 enzyme, which helps break down substances—including nicotine—in the bloodstream. By slowing this process, heptalactone may help keep the precious nicotine in your body longer.

Sugar

Burning sugar releases acetaldehyde (fermenting alcohol does the same thing). At least one study says acetaldehyde has a narcotic effect, which, if true, would be a very cost-effective thing to add to a cigarette. Acetaldehyde is also what scientists call a positive reinforcer: when it is combined with nicotine, each substance amplifies the other's effect on your brain (and the likelihood you'll want to keep smoking).

Levulinic Acid

This crystalline substance desensitizes the body's upper respiratory tract; if you inhale harsh substances (like smoke), this stuff leaves you with the perception of nothing but smoothness or mildness. It's also another way of juicing tobacco's high—levulinic acid enhances the binding of nicotine to the appropriate receptors in the brain, giving you more bang for the puff.

L-arginine

Smoking tobacco causes monocytes (specialized white blood cells) to stick to the endothelial cells on the inner walls of arteries and veins. This buildup, like all circulatory blockages, can lead to heart attack and stroke. Arginine, a common amino acid, may reverse some of this accumulation when taken orally. So, in a sense, maybe cigarettes aren't so bad after all.

Farnesol
A plant-based alcohol with a delicate floral scent, farnesol happens to inhibit the growth of some early cancer cells. This is no doubt added as a public service by the tobacco companies, since cigarettes don't cause cancer, right?

Isovaleric Acid
Imparts a cheesy or sweaty foot smell to cigarettes, which makes absolutely no sense from a marketing standpoint. But this stuff is also a pheromone found in the vaginal secretions of rhesus monkeys and is responsible for stimulating sexual response in males. Is this really a last-ditch attempt to make smoking sexy?

CIGARETTE LABELS

The top news story of 1964 was not the arrival of the Beatles in America, or the Freedom Riders fighting for civil rights in the South, or even President Johnson's landslide victory over Senator Barry Goldwater in that November's presidential election. It was the release on January 11 by US surgeon general Luther L. Terry of a report entitled "Smoking and Health," which showed "the strongest relationship between cigarette smoking and lung cancer" and "a very strong relationship, probably a causal relationship, between cigarette smoking and heart disease."

The report changed everything about how America (and eventually the world) viewed cigarettes. Congress sprang into action, creating federal guidelines for the sale, packaging, and advertising of cigarettes. Since 1965, cigarettes sold in the United States have had to have a warning label from the federal government, indicating—in many different phrases over the years—the hazards of smoking. And while these warnings have been credited with bringing down the rate of smoking in the US, why haven't they eradicated the habit completely?

An obscure 1973 tobacco company report may have the answer. Writing about the industry's need to gain new, younger smokers, R. J. Reynolds assistant director of research Claude Teague wrote:

> [A]t eighteen, one is immortal. Further, if the desire to be daring is part of the motivation to start smoking, the alleged risk of smoking may actually make smoking attractive. Finally, if the "older" establishment is preaching against smoking, the anti-establishment sentiment discussed above would cause the young to want to be defiant and smoke. Thus, a new brand aimed at the group should not in any way be promoted as a "health" brand, and perhaps should carry some implied risk. In this sense the warning label on the package may be a plus.

In other words, no good deed goes unpunished; the addition of a warning label might actually encourage certain people to smoke.

Coffee

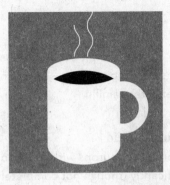

Cocainelike brain chemicals and the juice of death.

Caffeine

This white powder is why the world produces more than sixteen billion pounds of coffee beans per year. It's actually an alkaloid plant toxin (like nicotine and cocaine); plants use it to kill bugs. It stimulates us by blocking neuroreceptors for the sleep chemical adenosine. When the sleep chemical is blocked by caffeine, the result is you, awake.

Water

Hot H_2O is a super solvent, leaching flavors and oils out of the coffee bean. A good cup of joe is 98.75 percent water and 1.25 percent soluble plant matter. Caffeine is a diuretic, so coffee newbies pee out the water quickly; java junkies build up resistance.

2-Ethylphenol

This substance creates a tarlike, medicinal odor in your morning wake-up. Too much (in the range of one gram for every kilogram of body weight, far more than you'll get from a cup of coffee) makes rats stagger around their cages like the town drunk on New Year's Eve. It's also a component of cockroach alarm pheromones, chemical signals that warn the colony of danger.

Quinic Acid

That "sour coffee" burn in the pit of your stomach? This stuff. On the plus side, it's one of the starter chemicals in the formulation of flu-fighter Tamiflu.

3,5 Dicaffeoylquinic Acid

When scientists pretreat neurons with this acid in the lab, the cells are significantly (though not completely) protected from free-radical damage. Yup: coffee is a good source of antioxidants.

Dimethyl Disulfide

A natural product of roasting the green coffee bean, this compound is just at the threshold of detectability in brewed java. Good thing, too, as it's one of the compounds that gives human feces its odor.

Acetylmethylcarbinol

That rich, buttery taste in your daily jolt comes in part from this flammable yellow liquid, which helps give real butter its flavor and is a component of artificial flavoring in microwave popcorn.

Putrescine

Ever wonder what makes spoiled meat so poisonous? Here you go. Ptomaines like putrescine are produced when *E. coli* bacteria in the meat break down amino acids. Naturally present in coffee beans, it smells, as you might guess from the name, like Satan's outhouse.

Trigonelline

Chemically, it's a molecule of niacin with a methyl group attached. It breaks down into pyridines, which give coffee its sweet, earthy taste and also prevent the tooth-eating bacterium *Streptococcus mutans* from attaching to your teeth. Is there anything coffee can't do? It even fights the Cavity Creeps.

Niacin

A.k.a. vitamin B3. Trigonelline is unstable above 160 degrees Fahrenheit; at that temperature, the methyl group detaches, unleashing the niacin into your cup. Two or three espressos can provide half your recommended daily allowance.

Theophylline

One of the many chemical cousins of caffeine, this mild stimulant and muscle relaxant is used to relieve the symptoms of asthma, bronchitis, and emphysema. The downside? It can react badly with some of the newer antibiotics.

NATURAL

The FDA definition of "natural" is pretty freshman-level philo-sophical, to the point of analysis paralysis (it reads along the lines of "Once a food product has been harvested it is no longer fully 'natural' since it has been processed, even minimally, by hu-mans. So who can say what is 'natural' and what is not?"). Such a "Who are we to judge?" attitude doesn't really serve the public: if nothing is "natural," then the word has no legal meaning and therefore can be used however a food packager sees fit. So the FDA tempers their wishy-washiness with a carefully worded re-port of its past performance: "The agency has not objected to the use of the term if the food does not contain added color, artificial flavors, or synthetic substances." So, at best, that's all you can be *certain* "natural" means: no dyes, no artificial flavors, no plastic.

[BACKSTORY]

Coffee addiction is the developed world's second-most prevalent back monkey (after nicotine). Songs have been written about it, from Johann Sebastian Bach's *Coffee Cantata* to Julian Smith's "Racist Coffee." Many people literally (the literal meaning of "literally") can't get through the day without it. It's no wonder why people *really* didn't like having coffee torn apart like this.

And it's also not surprising that few coffee producers offer the public any useful information about the chemicals in their brew. Nescafé and Starbucks, just to choose two examples at random, nearly completely gloss over the chemicals in coffee on their websites. Their PR people are even less helpful,

AMMONIA

You think you know what ammonia smells like? You can't handle what ammonia smells like! In undiluted form, ammonia (NH_3) can be used as a chemical weapon; that's how badass ammonia *really* is. This compound of one nitrogen atom and three hydrogen atoms is actually one of the most useful chemicals in the universe. As a fertilizer, it forces plants to grow larger and stronger, whether they want to or not. As an antiseptic it kills nearly every type of microorganism; not even Chuck Norris has that kind of kill ratio. It is found in gas clouds out in space and on most of the planets in our solar system. Ammonia is so versatile that astrobiologists have speculated that other life forms with a different biochemistry could use ammonia the way we use water. Here's the weird thing—ammonia is technically flammable, but you don't have to worry about its catching fire: the temperature of the ammonia flame is lower than ammonia's ignition temperature. In other words, it's very difficult to keep an ammonia fire going.

limiting their replies to things like "the finest coffee beans" and "pure filtered water."

To get deep down inside the coffee bean, you have to search deep down in the Internet. On the USDA's website, there is a section called the Agricultural Research Service (ARS). And deep within the ARS website, there is a section called the Germplasm Resources Information Network (GRIN). And deep within GRIN, there is what looks for all the world like a rogue web page, containing something called Dr. Duke's Phytochemical and Ethnobotanical Databases.

Not a *Doonesbury* gag, this is a complete database taken from Dr. James Duke's groundbreaking work *Handbook of Phytochemical Constituents of GRAS Herbs and Other Economic Plants*. Duke found over a thousand chemicals in coffee alone. Anything you want to know about the naturally occurring plant-based chemicals on the USDA's "Generally Regarded as Safe" list can probably be found in Dr. Duke's. Happy hunting!

Cool Whip

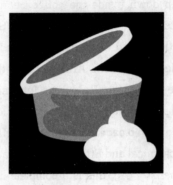

Synthetic wax + fats + sex grease = fake cream.

Water

It's the main ingredient. But like any whipped product, Cool Whip contains a high percentage of air. At forty-one cents per ounce, you're buying mostly water and air for just over twice what it would cost to whip real cream yourself.

Natural and Artificial Flavorings

Cool Whip doesn't really taste like much, but Kraft's recipe for blandness is a trade secret. That means the company doesn't have to disclose the specific flavorings.

Corn Syrup and High-Fructose Corn Syrup

Sugar by other names. Corn syrup is mostly glucose. High-fructose corn syrup is corn syrup treated with amylase and other enzymes, which together help convert glucose into fructose. A diet high in fructose is known to make research animals fatter than other diets, so keep your lab mice away from Cool Whip.

Hydrogenated Coconut and Palm Kernel Oil

Cool Whip needs to feel like whipped cream in the mouth without actually being, you know, made with cream. One cheap, reliable way to replicate the texture is by using semi-solidified plant oils. The best method of solidifying plant oils? Bubble high-pressure hydrogen through them. Of course, if not done completely, the result is trans fat. These days, Kraft avoids that.

Polysorbate 60

Polysorbates are made by polymerizing ethylene oxide (a precursor to antifreeze) with a sugar alcohol derivative. The result can be a detergent, an emulsifier, or, in the case of polysorbate 60, a major ingredient in some sexual lubricants.

Sodium Caseinate

Also common in powdered nondairy creamer, this protein derived from cow milk helps oil and water mix. The whole thing seems like a bizarre attempt to manufacture cream by extraterrestrials who have never actually tasted cream but know its chemical makeup.

Sorbitan Monostearate

Chemists call this stuff synthetic wax, and it's sometimes used as a hemorrhoid cream. It's one of the magical substances that keep Cool Whip from turning to liquid over time in the fridge.

Xanthan and Guar Gums

These are natural thickeners, and together they provide more viscosity than either does alone. Guar also helps retard the formation of ice crystals, allowing Cool Whip to remain frozen for months and still maintain its whipped fluffiness.

[BACKSTORY]

In 2007, *Wired* got its own TV show on PBS. Called *Wired Science*, it was hosted by the actor/comedian/nerd Chris Hardwick. I was honored when they told me they wanted to present my articles as a special segment of the show.

The format was simple: Chris Hardwick stood at a long table loaded with ingredients. He'd present each ingredient to the audience, explain what it did, and challenge them to try to figure out what well-known product all the ingredients added up to. At the end, Chris would then reveal the product.

The first product he ever did was Cool Whip, using this write-up as a template. And from the very beginning we were causing trouble for PBS. Go online and watch the PBS video of Chris Hardwick deconstructing Cool Whip (which for a while was the most viewed PBS video online ever) at https://www.youtube.com/watch?v=PcRF8HYvj2A.

Watch carefully between 1:30 and 1:33 in the video. There's an extremely awkward cut in the video, and lo and

---

CARBOHYDRATE

What's the difference between a carbohydrate and a hydrocarbon, aside from the fact that one is edible and the other is motor oil? A hydrocarbon is just what its name implies: hydrogen and carbon, and nothing else. A carbohydrate, on the other hand, is carbon that has been *hydrated*, that is, has had water's constituent atoms added to it, with the result that a carbohydrate is made of carbon, hydrogen, and oxygen. Take glucose, whose chemical formula is $C_6H_{12}O_6$. For a long time scientists thought its makeup was actually $C_6\text{-}H_2O\text{-}H_2O\text{-}H_2O$. In addition to being a food source, carbohydrates are also structural elements like wood and cotton, as well as the backbone of DNA and RNA.

behold, there's suddenly a new ingredient on the table that Chris hasn't talked about. Is he going to talk about it later? Nope; by the end of the video there are clearly ten items on the table, but Chris only talked about nine of them.

The item removed during that awkward edit, the item Chris never got to talk about on TV, was sexual lubricant. PBS apparently had absolutely no problem deconstructing an iconic American commercial product. They had no problem with the sarcasm Chris used in the piece. But the very idea of showing and broadcasting (or even mentioning) actual sexual lubricant on PBS was a little too frightening for them. Apparently the last thing they needed was Senator Moron from the great state of Moronica to make a speech about the "filth and perversion" PBS was putting into their science shows. Better to pretend the sexual lubricant never happened than to risk that.

Chris Hardwick continued to do the segment, presenting different products, for the entirety of the show's thirteen-week run. My personal favorite: when he brought the actor Rainn Wilson out to guess the contents of NyQuil.

Doritos Late Night All Nighter Cheeseburger Chips

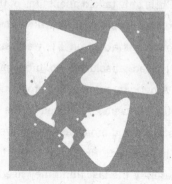

Armpit bacteria, fake tomatoes, and little bits of gold.

Whole Corn

The word "*doritos*" is supposedly pidgin Spanish for "little bits of gold." The main ingredient in these bits of gold is heated and steeped in an alkaline solution, usually lye or lime. This frees up the corn's niacin and restructures some of its amino acids, leading to better protein quality.

Vegetable Oil

Each chip is nearly 29 percent fat by weight, and almost all of that is corn oil, sunflower oil, or soybean oil. That's good, because fat activates the brain's natural mu-opioid receptors, provoking what scientists call a hedonic response; you want to eat more fat, which makes a stronger hedonic response, which makes you want to eat more fat, and . . . dude, don't bogart the bag!

Milk

Simple pasteurized cow milk, used as the basis for the two cheeses.

Cheddar Cheese Cultures

Usually *Lactococcus lactis cremoris* bacteria. They're injected into the milk during the cheese-making process, and their enzymes break down milk proteins into various smelly/tasty compounds.

Monosodium Glutamate

Some people swear they can taste ketchup on these chips, even though tomatoes aren't on the ingredient list. Since the principal component of a tomato's flavor is glutamic acid, it is possible (Frito-Lay isn't talking) that the addition of MSG and a few spices is responsible for the crypto-ketchup taste sensation.

Salt

The *Diagnostic and Statistical Manual of Mental Disorders* lists seven criteria, any three of which make a substance addictive. Salt meets four of them: withdrawal symptoms, the development of tolerance, inability to control level of usage, and difficulty quitting or restricting (even with full knowledge of health hazards).

Sugar

The last piece of the unholy trinity: fat, salt, sugar. Lab rats given sugar show an increase in their brain's D1 (excitatory) receptors and a decrease in D2 (inhibitory) receptors. Just like lab rats given cocaine! Over time, they need more and more of the white stuff—either sugar or blow—to get the buzz.

Natural Beef Flavor

If you pressure-cook clarified beef stock and then distill away the water, you're left with chemicals like 4-hydroxy-5-methyl-3(2H)-furanone, 2-methyl-3-furanthiol, and bis(2-methyl-3-furyl) disulfide. All the flavor of a hamburger with none of the nutrition.

Swiss Cheese Cultures

Those bubble holes in Swiss cheese? The acne sores on your face? They're both the result of gas and acids given off by members of the *Propionibacterium* family, which have been distilled into these chips.

. . . .

Corn Maltodextrin

This is glucose that is going through a period of identity confusion. Not exactly starch and not exactly sugar, maltodextrin is legally defined as a chain of glucose molecules with a dextrose equivalency rating of less than 20 (corn syrup is 68, starch is 0). Different kinds of maltodextrin can be used as a fat substitute or fiber supplement, but here its absorptive qualities and lack of taste are put to use as a medium for delivering the beef and cheese flavors to your mouth.

. . . .

Onion Powder

Onions complete the cheeseburger—their sulfurous goodness strengthens the savory flavor of the meaty compounds.

. . . .

Mustard Seed Powder

What's a cheeseburger without mustard? But the most common complaint about this snack is that Frito-Lay went too heavy on the stuff. It's so hard to fake things just right.

. . . .

[BACKSTORY]

I was in my local Target when I first came across this bag. Cheeseburger-flavored Doritos? How did they manage to do that? *Why* did they manage to do that? Did people write letters to Frito-Lay saying, "You know, I like the Nacho and Cool Ranch flavors, but could you make something more cheeseburgery?" Did it come from a focus group Frito-Lay held with college stoners? "Dude, sometimes we want cheeseburgers late at night, but, like, we don't want to go out and get food, so we just, like, eat Doritos. You know what would be awesome? If you guys could like make Doritos that taste like cheeseburgers! That would be so awesome!" We'll probably never know.

There in the store, I read the ingredient list and my eyes lit up. At the time, Doritos Late Night All Nighter Cheeseburger chips were made with pork enzymes, to give them a unique flavor. Pork enzymes! Pork. Enzymes. Enzymes are necessary to turn milk into cheese, and traditionally those have been cow enzymes. But pork? I love working on those products that contain unexpected ingredients, and here was a great one—after all, you probably don't anticipate pork enzymes in your cheeseburger chips (although you probably should). More to the point, people who follow the kosher or halal dietary rules are forbidden to eat anything derived from pork. Would they notice the pork in these corn chips? Of course, people keeping kosher aren't supposed to be eating cheeseburgers either, but would that apply to something that simply *tasted* like the forbidden food?

Obviously, this pork enzyme thing was something I had to speak to the folks at Doritos about. Frito-Lay, the makers

EAFUS

This acronym stands for "Everything Added to Food in the United States." It's a database of 3,968 (as of this writing) ingredients and additives that are (or have been) legally permitted to be used in food in the US. It is used by just about anyone hoping to introduce a new food product to the American people. It is currently divided into six subcategories:

A. Fully up-to-date toxicology information is available (or has been requested) for the substance. The vast majority of EAFUS substances fall into this category.

B. Banned: The substance was once allowed in food but has since been banned. Things like cyclamate artificial sweetener (banned in 1969 as a suspected carcinogen) and Red Dye #2 (banned in 1976, same reason). This is the smallest category in EAFUS.

C. New: The substance is being used in food, and the FDA toxicology reports are in progress. Contrary to popular belief, food manufacturers don't necessarily have to clear new food additives with the FDA in advance.

D. NIL: The substance has been listed as an additive in the past, but there is currently no reported use of the substance in food. However, toxicology information is still available. This category includes such wonder substances as ferrous carbonate, an iron supplement used to remedy tired blood (available in pills, tablets, and gelatin capsules), and sweet wormwood extract.

E. NUL: There is no reported use of the substance and there is no toxicology data (however, the substance is still on the EAFUS list). This mystery category includes substances like hydrolyzed milk protein, a relatively harmless extract that is used in cosmetics but not in foods, and acrolein, a thick, oily gasoline residue the CDC has declared toxic.

F. Everything else: These are substances that are being used in foods, but no toxicology reports have yet been ordered by the FDA. This is real Wild West territory: it includes food additives like caprolactam, a precursor chemical to nylon; methionyl butyrate, an artificial flavor; and grapefruit juice.

of Doritos, is owned by PepsiCo ("A leading global food and beverage company with brands that are respected household names throughout the world"). After finally reaching the right person, I asked them point-blank about the pork enzymes that can be found in the ingredient list. "What were they used for?" I asked. "What was special about pork enzymes that could not be handled by other types of enzymes?" The person at PepsiCo said he would get back to me.

Now repeat that several times over the next several weeks: I would call PepsiCo, I'd ask some questions about the pork enzymes, they would tell me that they'd have to get back to me, we would say good-bye. One day, I called them up, fully expecting to go through the same Kabuki theater we had been playing for the past weeks. Instead, the person I spoke to feigned complete innocence of any knowledge of pork enzymes. I told them I was calling about the pork enzymes in Doritos Late Night All Nighter Cheeseburger chips. They told me there were no pork enzymes in Doritos Late Night All Nighter Cheeseburger chips. I told them that there were. They told me there weren't. I promised to call back.

I went to the store and grabbed a bag of chips. There were no pork enzymes listed. Later, while I was actually researching this article, a Frito-Lay spokesperson confirmed that pork enzymes had been part of Doritos but were no longer in use. Was my persistent questioning the reason for the change? I strongly doubt that I had anything to do with Frito-Lay's abandoning the use of pork enzymes; that move was probably in the pipeline for months before I came along. No matter; there were still loads about this product to write about.

I contacted a different person at Frito-Lay/PepsiCo to ask some more general questions about Doritos. No problem, he said, Doritos is all natural, we have no secrets. I started to list my questions, when he interrupted me to say that it would be much better if I e-mailed him the questions so he could do some research and be sure he got the best possible answers to me. "Unless you're trying to trick me with some 'gotcha' questions over the phone, ha ha," he added. We both shared a sarcastic laugh. I e-mailed him seven questions. Ten days later he responded:

1. The answer to this is proprietary.
2. Yes, little bits of gold.
3. The answer to this is proprietary.
4. The answer to this is proprietary.
5. The answer to this is proprietary.
6. Yes, pasteurized.
7. The answer to this is proprietary.

That was the extent of their assistance. The rest of the piece came from my own research. A few weeks later, when the story was done, I contacted the same guy to let him know that he would be hearing from our fact-checkers, to verify the two answers he gave us and some other things we had researched. He was astounded. How *dare* we write a story about PepsiCo when PepsiCo stopped cooperating with us? I told him we're journalists—that's what we do for a living. He told us it was *very* irresponsible for us as journalists to write an article about a company that didn't want to be written about. And especially without opening a dialogue with the company giving them a chance to tell their side of the story! I firmly believe this man will head PepsiCo someday.

Easy Cheese Aerosol Spread

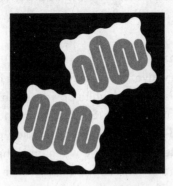

Our new slogan: Just enough cheese to meet federal guidelines.

Whey

The cheese-making process removes 80 to 90 percent of milk's moisture, some of which is in the form of liquidy whey proteins. This by-product is usually thrown out, but Kraft plows it back into Easy Cheese to increase volume (it is, in other words, filler)—and passes the savings along to you.

Canola Oil

Unlike most other cheeses, this one has to move. A generous amount of this oil keeps the cheese from solidifying.

Salt

Increases the osmotic transport of moisture, so it inhibits bacterial growth—in other words, it's a preservative. Easy Cheese has twice the sodium of typical organic cheddar.

Sodium Citrate

The sodium in this compound exchanges ions with the calcium in the milk and "softens" the water-soluble portion of the cheese, enabling it to mix thoroughly with the fat-soluble component. That's called emulsification. But this compound provides two bangs for the price of one: the citric-acid-derived citrate boosts the sour "bite" of cheddar flavor.

Sodium Phosphate

Degreaser, preservative, urine acidifier, enema ingredient—is there anything this family of white powders can't do? Here, it's another emulsifying agent. Since sodium phosphate was a component of old-fashioned embalming fluids, proponents of natural cheese cited this additive when lobbying to have Kraft's products regulated as "embalmed cheese." The Feds settled on the less-mortifying "process cheese."

Calcium Phosphate

Sodium phosphate tends to block up the calcium in cheese, making it unavailable to the body. So it's possible that calcium phosphate has to be added to make Easy Cheese healthier. It also makes it legal for Kraft to label every can "an excellent source of calcium."

Lactic Acid

Bacteria, either found naturally in milk or added in the cheese-making process, digest the milk sugar lactose and produce lactic acid. It tastes a little sour, because that's how your taste buds interpret hydrogen ions, a key component of every acid.

Sodium Alginate

Nearly every good processed food has seaweed extract, and Easy Cheese is no exception. Alginate, a gum found in the cell walls of brown algae, is flavorless but increases viscosity.

Apocarotenal

This yellow-orange pigment, found in spinach and citrus fruits, enhances the color of processed cheese.

. . . .

The Can

Easy Cheese is not a true aerosol—the food never comes in contact with propellant. The can has two sections: the bottom is filled with nitrogen gas, and the top with cheese. Press the nozzle and the nitrogen pressure pushes the cheese out of the can. The nozzle is notched for two reasons: to produce those pretty little floret patterns when the cheese is released, and to ensure that the tasty condiment comes out even if the end of the nozzle is pushed right up against the cracker.

. . . .

[BACKSTORY]

The first product I ever investigated!

While Easy Cheese will never be mistaken for health food, it isn't quite the industrial slurry some think it is. About 100 years ago, itinerant cheese peddler James L. Kraft pasteurized some shredded cheddar cheese, added sodium phosphate as an emulsifier, and sold the result as "process cheese," a safe cheese that sliced easily and wouldn't spoil in those primitive, unrefrigerated days. With slight variations, as new chemicals have been discovered, the recipe has been pretty much unchanged since then.

One can contains seven 32-gram servings of Easy Cheese. Since most cheese eaters can't tell a 32-gram serving by sight, it's really up to you how many squirts you get. Eating one full can of Easy Cheese (handily within the skill set of the average American couch potato) provides all the sodium, all the calcium, and half the cholesterol you should eat in one day. To put it another way, after a single can of Easy Cheese you're pretty much limited to bread and water for the next 24 hours, if you want to stay within the recommended daily intake guidelines.

The can is marked A GOOD SOURCE OF CALCIUM, and thanks to some additional ingredients, it is. The can also brags that Easy Cheese is made from Real Cheese. Put there to reassure fortysomething Yuppie baby mamas, who no doubt think Easy Cheese is made from radioactive dioxin. In reality, all process cheese is made from real cheese, if you go far enough back in the production process.

Not bragged about, but printed on the can in eye-squinting

CHEESE, PROCESSED CHEESE, CHEESE FOOD, CHEESE SPREAD

One of the bravest humans in prehistory was the person who first ate cheese. Imagine it: they had probably recently discovered the art of using an eviscerated cow stomach as a small storage vessel. When they poured milk into that vessel, they had no idea that the naturally occurring enzymes in the stomach, collectively called rennet, would go to work coagulating the milk, beginning the process of turning it into cheese. What would you do if your morning milk had suddenly turned into a smelly lump of curds and whey? Yes, it took great courage to take that first bite.

Since then, cheese-making has been a widely practiced art. In warmer climates, cheeses tended to be softer, with more curd: ricotta, feta, and jibneh are the best examples. In the cooler climates of Europe, cheese-making required less salt, which allowed various bacteria and molds to infiltrate the cheese, leading to the sharply flavored cheddars, the moldy Roqueforts, and the bubbly Swiss cheeses.

And then there's American cheese. American is what is known as a "processed cheese"—that is, a cheese that does not exist in nature, but is instead manufactured by mixing, with the aid of heat, one or more cheeses of the same or different varieties, along with chemical emulsifiers, into what the Code of Federal Regulations calls "a homogeneous plastic mass," which is poured into a mold and allowed to cool. The moisture and fat content of the resulting cheese must be within 1 percent of the average of the base cheeses, and various preservatives, coloring agents, and unfermented milk solids can be added.

But that's nothing compared to "cheese food." Isn't cheese *already* food? According to the USDA, cheese food is processed cheese without all that cheese. Specifically, cheese food can be made from only 51 percent cheese; the rest of the weight can be made from cream, buttermilk, cheese whey, anhydrous milk fat, dehydrated cream, albumin from cheese whey, lecithin, and skim milk cheese.

And finally, there's cheese spread. In most cases, cheese spread is cheese food with a higher moisture content and lower fat, which makes it more easily spreadable. Since this combination is unstable, cheese food almost always includes extra emulsifiers and stabilizers to keep it from separating.

tiny type, is Easy Cheese's Federal HAZMAT rating: DOT2P. This Department of Transportation code indicates that a pressurized can of Easy Cheese is nonexplosive and can withstand an internal pressure of 131 psi at 54.4 degrees Celsius before bursting.

Also: You know that little rubber button on the bottom of the can? It is the fill valve, and it also serves as a relief valve if the can is stored in a hot place (or in a fire), which might otherwise cause the can to burst.

Enfamil Baby Formula

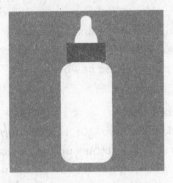

Milk, vitamins, and a dollop of parental guilt.

Nonfat Milk

To a first approximation, all mammals produce pretty much the same milk: an emulsion of saturated fats, proteins, and sugars in water. The difference is in the details, in the specific components and their percentages. Straight cow milk is great for li'l Bossy but not for little Bradley. Human newborns can't always use cow milk's particular fat efficiently: up to 50 percent goes right through them. What's more, bovine proteins can wreak havoc in the infant gut, leading to allergies. Removing the fat and heat-treating these proteins is the first step in turning cow milk into faux human milk.

Lactose

The actual milk sugar molecule is the same whether it comes from an udder or a breast. However, human milk contains more natural lactose than cow milk. To sweeten the deal, formula makers add extra lactose, which breaks down into the simpler carbohydrates glucose and galactose.

Palm Olein Oil

Palmitic acid makes up 20 to 24 percent of the fat in human milk, so Enfamil supplements its formula with palm olein oil. But that switcheroo doesn't always work. The slightly different arrangement of triglycerides causes constipation in many formula-fed babies. Palm olein also tends to produce the infamous "yellow poop" of the newborn.

Mortierella Alpina Oil

Extracted from *Mortierella* fungus, this oil supplies arachidonic acid. Bodybuilders use AA to bulk up their muscles. Infants use it to bulk up their neurons, because AA is the principal omega-6 fatty acid in the brain. It's also a precursor of eicosanoids, hormones that play a role in numerous functions, including blood clotting.

Nucleotides

Wait a minute: nucleotides are the building blocks of DNA. Is this an insidious program of the genetic manipulation of the next generation through their infant formula? Not quite. When cells are damaged, they can release these compounds, cuing the immune system to start cleaning house. Adding them to infant formula jump-starts a baby's antibody response to immunization. Plus, they may help put the kid to sleep.

Ferrous Sulfate

$FeSO_4$ is among the best-absorbed iron compounds, but it has to be balanced precisely: too much iron in the diet leads to the infamous "green poop" of the newborn.

L-carnitine

In adults, this nutrient shows potential to treat congestive heart failure, lower triglycerides, and boost sperm count. Since babies don't have to worry about any of those things, they use this stuff to metabolize fats.

. . . .

Crypthecodinium Cohnii Oil

This oil is rich in docosahexaenoic acid, or DHA, which until recently US infant formulas lacked. The long-chain fatty acid is essential to the development of a newborn's brain and visual systems, and seems to increase information processing in infants; babies without adequate levels of DHA can be less curious and slower to get the point.

. . . .

Inositol

It's an enzyme activator, a cell growth factor, and a component of cell membranes. Breast milk is loaded with the stuff, so it makes sense to put inositol in formula. But studies of preemies show that the formula version doesn't last as long in the bloodstream.

. . . .

Choline Chloride

A.k.a. vitamin B4. Provides choline, which is essential for organ growth in neonates. Human milk usually provides it in the form of glycerophosphocholine, but that costs about one hundred times as much per gram as choline chloride, and new parents have enough expenses.

. . . .

[BACKSTORY]

Ohhhhhhhh boy. Do not make parents freak out about their children. They will hurt you badly.

If you think about it, so many consumer products are nothing more than attempts to artificially re-create something that already exists—usually in abundance. There's no worldwide shortage of whipped cream, yet someone actually went through all the trouble to brainstorm, experiment, test, package, and market Cool Whip. Neither is there a shortage of orange juice, butter, or human tears, and yet SunnyD, I Can't Believe It's Not Butter, and Visine sit on our shelves.

So it shouldn't be a surprise that the most intimate human exchange—a mother feeding herself to her baby—has been synthesized. Human babies have been swallowing human milk for as long as humans have existed, and no food is better for them. So why does baby formula even exist?

One reason is that there are some situations where mothers

CHOLESTEROL

Cholesterol is the steroid no one wants to abuse. Actually, cholesterol is one of the most vital compounds of life, since it makes up most of our cell membranes, the things that keep our cells together. Without cholesterol, we'd all just be giant puddles of undifferentiated protoplasm. (More than we already are, I mean.) The problem is that too much of a specific type of cholesterol can result in the formation of atheromas—globules of cholesterol, fatty acids, calcium, and connective tissue—inside our arteries. If the atheromas get too big, they can effectively cut off the flow of blood through the artery. Since arteries are the main vessels supplying oxygenated blood all over the body, blocking them in this way is never a good thing.

simply can't produce milk, or enough milk, or they are otherwise prevented from nursing. For them, formula can literally be a lifesaver.

But there's a flip side. In the 1970s western companies aggressively encouraged mothers in the developing world to switch to baby formula instead of breast-feeding. Like any other advertising campaign, baby formula was touted as a way into "the good life": simple and convenient, formula would make babies strong while also enabling mothers to go back to work. A win-win for all, right? The companies capped their sales pitch by giving away generous free samples—sometimes even in the hospital. The free samples were just large enough to last until the mother's milk dried up. At that point, the family had no choice in the matter—they were locked into buying formula until the baby was weaned.

While formula advertising practices have changed, it's hard to see how any lab-based concoction will be better for a baby than its own mother's milk. At least until we've got cage after cage of orangutans genetically engineered to produce human milk.

And you know someone's got to be working on that.

Enzyte

Insert "Insert dick joke here" here.

L-arginine

It's no surprise that Enzyte's "natural male enhancement" supplement—with its late-night TV ads aimed right at the male psyche—would feature this amino acid. L-arginine is a natural precursor to nitric oxide (NO), and nitric oxide is the potent vasodilator that puts the "erect" in "erection." Nitric oxide opens the vascular floodgates, allowing blood to swell into the *corpus cavernosum* and *corpus spongiosum* of the penis, thereby making an erection. But while NO deficiency might prevent an erection, overcharging the system with excess levels of nitric oxide to "enhance" an erection doesn't work—the body simply adjusts to the new NO levels and maintains the same response.

Horny Goat Weed

The hardy Asian plants of the genus *Epimedium* produce icariin, a flavonoid that inhibits expression of the PDE5 family of enzymes. So what, you say? Well, PDE5 prevents erections. (Stifling PDE5 is Viagra's entire raison d'être.) If you knock out the thing that's preventing an erection, the thinking goes, you cause an erection. A study at Zhejiang Chinese Medical

University claimed that icariin also increases short-term production of nitric oxide. If true, we all know what *that* means.

Zinc

Zinc deficiency in the diet of preadolescent boys can result in decreased genital growth. In grown men, low zinc intake correlates with low testosterone and low semen output. Low semen doesn't directly have anything to do with the ability to get an erection, but remember; Enzyte is all about *male enhancement,* and that almost certainly includes the bullets as well as the gun. However, if you have normal Zn levels, it won't necessarily spike your cocktail; in fact, bingeing on the metal can lead to reduced immune function.

Tribulus terrestris

No, it's not the juice of a *Star Trek* furry; it's a weedy flowering plant used as an Ayurvedic aphrodisiac (the Enzyte people are leaving no culture unrepresented). Studies have indicated that protodioscin, a steroidal saponin found in the *Tribulus* fruit, stimulates production of male hormones and nitric oxide; however, at least one other study shows that it doesn't. The real trouble with *Tribulus* is that overuse has been linked to kidney and liver poisoning.

Korean Red Ginseng

Traditional Chinese medicine claims that Asian ginseng promotes yang, the masculine life force. Traditional Western medicine shows that steroidlike components called ginsenosides promote production of nitric oxide, the erection's "life force." A 2007 Brazilian study asserted that ginseng raised rigidity and penetration scores. (Yes, there's a five-step protocol for gauging erections.) But don't get too cocksure: a Korean study subsequently threw cold water on those findings.

Avena sativa Extract

Wilford Brimley was right: eat your *Avena sativa* (a.k.a. oatmeal). Multiple studies have shown that whole grains like oatmeal can lower blood pressure, which *might* make more blood available to the penis.

. . . .

Copper

Enzyte provides 200 percent of your FDA daily recommended intake of copper. Clinical copper deficiency is uncommon in humans, but it can cause a decrease in nitric oxide. Still, since too much Cu is a risk factor for cardiovascular disease as well as related erectile dysfunction, if you're adamant about wanting to use copper to raise your flag, instead of Enzyte you should put a ring on it.

. . . .

My preferred style of comedy is what I think of as a Benchleyesque dry wit. (You the reader will have to decide if I reach that level of skill; I know that I certainly aim for that.) The point is: I don't really do dick jokes. And yet, when the opportunity presented itself, in the form of Enzyte "male enhancement" capsules, how could I resist? There are probably more penis and/or erection jokes in this one piece than I've told in the past three years. And the amazing thing is how easily they popped up.

See what I did there?

I actually learned so much while doing this story. As you know, an erection is caused by letting blood flow into reservoirs in the penis. These swollen tissues naturally pinch off the veins leading out of the penis, thus maintaining an erection until the situation is resolved.

Erection problems relating to blood flow should therefore be solved by using vasodilators: drugs that open up the blood vessels, letting more blood in. The problem is that by indiscriminately opening all types of blood vessels, such vasodilators let blood in, but they also let blood right back out again.

Viagra's trick is that it opens the penile arteries, letting blood in, and closes the penile veins, thereby *keeping* blood in. And it appears that there are herbs and such in Enzyte that have the same selective function. Viagra does this by stopping the breakdown of nitric oxide. Since the penis (and clitoris) are very sensitive to nitric oxide concentrations, not removing nitric oxide leads to longer physical signs of arousal. The amyl nitrate "poppers" that people used in the

SOURCES

"A excellent source of X" means the product contains 20 percent or more of the daily recommended requirement of X. Synonyms are "High in X" and "Rich in X."

"A good source of X" means the product contains between 10 and 19 percent of the daily recommended requirement of X. Synonyms are "Provides X" and "Contains X."

"Enriched with X" means the product contains at least 10 percent more of X than it would normally have. A product that normally provides ten grams of protein could be "enriched" to provide eleven grams. Synonyms are "More," "Fortified with," "Extra," "Plus," and "Added."

"High Potency" means the product contains 100 percent of the daily recommended intake of X. Vitamin supplements, if they contain the full daily requirement of the vitamin, are by definition "high potency." Multivitamins must specify which vitamins are at 100 percent: "One A Day with High Potency Vitamin E" would simply mean the pill contained all the vitamin E you needed that day. It says nothing about the quality of the vitamin.

"Zero": If the serving contains less than 0.5 gram of something (such as fats, carbohydrates, protein, fiber), the content may be expressed as zero. Amounts less than five calories may be expressed as zero. Products that contain less than two milligrams of cholesterol in a serving may state the cholesterol content as zero.

And the most damning: according to federal regulations [21CFR101.9(b)(1)], the total serving size of a product is the "amount of food customarily consumed per eating occasion by persons 4 years of age." Why is serving size based on the amount a four-year-old can eat, and not like, say, a normal adult human being? Because, according to an FDA spokesperson, "That's around the time the child moves from toddler food to adult food." If that answer makes logical sense to you, you may have a future in the exciting field of government regulation.

seventies to get high (and to cause/maintain an erection) exploited this phenomenon; the body converted the nitrate to nitric oxide, which then did its work.

The problem is, of course (as you know, said the professor) that pinching off any vein—thus decreasing blood flow—for more than a few hours is asking for all sorts of trouble. This is why any male erection drug tells you to run screaming to the emergency room if your erection lasts more than four hours. I think I saw the phrases "oxygen-deprived tissue necrosis" and "formation of scar tissue" and "permanent loss of function" in the literature, but I really can't swear to it, as I got so freaked out I had to keep shutting down the computer and going for a walk.

I ended the piece by saying that one way to maintain an erection is to "put a ring on it." I'm talking, of course, about the sexual aid known as the cock ring (or, more gently, "erection ring" or "tension ring"). It's simply a mechanical means of blocking the penile veins, thus trapping the blood in the penis and maintaining an erection.

The thing is, when you do an Internet search for the terms "zinc," "copper," and "erection," you don't just get information on Enzyte and other herbal-type remedies. You also get information about the zinc/copper cock ring.

The zinc/copper cock ring works on a totally different principle than other cock rings. The zinc/copper cock ring turns the penis into a battery. I say again, *a cock ring made of zinc and copper turns the penis into a battery*. A conductive solution, in the form of salty sweat, between two different metals will cause electrons to flow from one side to the other. A lot depends on the salt content of the sweat, but under the right conditions the two metals can produce 1.5 volts, as much as a D cell. So the penis keeps going . . . and going . . . and going. . . .

(I know, this stuff just writes itself.)

Fun fact: the blood pressure of an erect penis can sometimes be as high as fifteen to twenty points above the patient's standard blood pressure. How did they measure this? With a tiny one-inch-wide blood pressure cuff, of course.

Hostess Lemon Fruit Pie

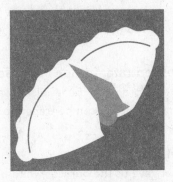

Enjoy sweet lemony goodness on the way to your angioplasty.

Agar

Remember back in high school biology class, when you cultured bacteria on an agar medium in petri dishes? This is the same stuff. It's actually a gelatinous preparation of the cell walls of red algae, used to thicken the fruit filling. On ingredient labels, it's sometimes called red seaweed, likely because the idea of ingesting seaweed is somewhat palatable (think sushi). Eating red algae, on the other hand, is totally disgusting.

High-Fructose Corn Syrup, Corn Syrup, Sugar

It wouldn't be a proper snack food if it didn't have three types of sugar, would it? In fact, almost one-third of the total weight of a Lemon Fruit Pie comes from this trio of sweeteners.

Vegetable and/or Animal Shortening

One of the paradoxes of the kitchen is that you can't produce light, flaky, delicate crusts if you don't use the thickest, heaviest shortening. And in industrial quantities, producing pastries with butter is right out, since the water in butter can make pastry tough and chewy. Which type of shortening is used in these pies depends on the state of the commodities market. Your scrumptious treat could be made with soybean oil today, but if the price of bulk shortening changes tomorrow, nothing goes better with the zesty taste of lemon than . . . beef fat. Yup, your Fruit Pie might be fluffed with ol' Bossy's blubber.

Lemon Juice Concentrate, Lemon Juice Solid, Lemon Oil

Finally, some fruit. According to the label, only about 7 percent or less of this Lemon Fruit Pie can be traced to lemons.

Enriched Wheat Flour

The ingredient that gave us the phrase "white-bread America." The first standards for enriching bread were set by the US in 1941, suggesting (and later requiring) the addition of iron and the B vitamins thiamine, riboflavin, and niacin (and later, folic acid) to white wheat flour. The result? Baby boomers grew up as the healthiest American generation in history. And now? Wheat plantings in the US are down nearly one-third since the 1980s, mostly due to decreased demand for wheat from, among other people, baby boomers. White flour's somewhat tarnished reputation makes it perfect for junktastic foods like Fruit Pies.

Locust Bean Gum

An extract of the seeds of the carob tree, locust bean gum was known to the ancient Egyptians, who used it to bind the wrappings of mummies. Here it is used for somewhat the same purpose: it keeps the crust from getting soggy and letting the fruity goodness leak out.

Calcium Sulfate

Plaster of Paris. Used for millennia to congeal soy milk into tofu, this gunk has hundreds of applications—many a school science project (like a baking soda and vinegar volcano) was modeled in plaster of Paris. In a Fruit Pie, it may be present as a coagulant, as a gel extender (helping to hold the moisture in), or just to add calcium.

. . . .

Artificial Flavor

Hostess won't say what it uses. But most citrus flavors can be derived from naturally occurring terpenes, plant-based hydrocarbons that can be replicated easily in the lab by distilling the mother lode of terpenes: turpentine.

. . . .

ORGANIC (FOODS)

As the USDA sees it, "organic" is a process, not a thing: a production management system that promotes and enhances biodiversity, biological cycles, soil biological activity, and ecological harmony, based on minimal use of "off-farm inputs" such as conventional pesticides, fertilizers made with synthetic ingredients or sewage sludge, bioengineering, or ionizing radiation. It says nothing about the nutritional content of the resulting food; you can easily grow low-quality food in a totally organic way. It also doesn't guarantee that other outside contaminants haven't entered the food, nor does it promise that the food hasn't been adulterated after it left the farm. Simply put, "organic" does not (and according to the USDA, *cannot*) ensure that products are completely free of residue.

Turpentine? The horrible smelly paint thinner, that turpentine? One of the ingredients in a Fruit Pie may very well be a derivative of paint thinner?

Actually, it is not as bad as it sounds. Nearly all plant flavors—from oranges to peaches to tomatoes to rutabagas—come from combining only a handful of naturally produced chemicals. It just so happens that turpentine is a hodgepodge of many of those chemicals. To make lemon flavor, you can simply start with turpentine and remove all the chemicals that aren't in lemons. You end up with something that is chemically identical to something extracted from a lemon but that came from a pine tree. Artificial orange and almond flavors, as well as citronella and lilac and many others, can also be synthesized from turpentine. The interesting thing is that, say, the plant-based octyl acetate you get from oranges is exactly the same plant-based octyl acetate you get from turpentine, yet one from oranges is deemed natural and the one from pine is artificial.

This is one of those items where you look at the ingredient list and say, "You really don't want to know. No, you *really* don't want to know."

Hot Pockets Pepperoni Pizza

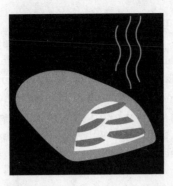

It can't be real pizza with imitation cheese,
but no one thinks this is real pizza.

Unbleached Enriched Flour

Is there bleach in some types of flour? Sort of—substances like chlorine (in tiny amounts) can be used to turn the normally beige-brown flour snowy white. The popularity of bleached flour products in America after World War II led to what detractors call the "white bread" homogeneity of the 1950s. Yet unbleached flour can still be whitish in color, because simply letting freshly milled grain sit for several weeks enables oxygen in the air to go to work on the wheat's naturally occurring pigments (called xanthophylls), oxidizing them from yellowish to white. Because the flour also has niacin, iron, and various B vitamins added to it, it is also described as "enriched."

Pepperoni

Technically, pepperoni is a variety of salami, a dry sausage that can be stored at room temperature ("shelf-stable," as they say in the food industry). It is loaded with sodium, which draws the water out of the meat, making the internal environment too dry for bacterial growth. Pepperoni can be made of almost any meat; Hot Pockets uses a mixture of pork and beef.

Imitation Mozzarella Cheese

Is this some vat-grown silicone/plastic that jiggles like real moozadel'? Of course not: imitation mozzarella actually contains mozzarella cheese, just not enough of it to actually be called real mozzarella. Most of the imitation cheese by weight is made of things like milk, food starch, lactic acid, and gum made from the fronds of red seaweed. With a tiny bit of real mozzarella cheese buried deep inside.

Tomato Paste

Tomato juice, tomato sauce, and tomato paste are all more or less macerated tomatoes without the seeds and skin; the difference between the three lies in their water content. In Italy, really old-fashioned tomato paste is made by letting pureed tomatoes dry in the summer sun. In the industrialized food wastes of North America, tomato paste is much wetter, but still dryer than tomato juice or sauce.

Partially Hydrogenated Soybean Oil

Hydrogenation, as applied here, refers to the art of bubbling pressurized hydrogen gas through a liquid—in this case, soybean oil. Some of the hydrogen will attach itself to the carbon chains in the soybean oil molecules, making the oil more *saturated* (with hydrogen), and thus raising its melting point so that it remains solid at room temperature. The problem is that in the hydrogenation process, some of the soybean oil may be converted from healthy *cis* fats, which your body needs, into unhealthy *trans* fats, which your body most emphatically doesn't need.

Calcium Sulfate

Plaster of Paris, remember? This white powder is commonly used in baked goods that might be frozen before they are eaten. It serves as a drying agent to keep the Hot Pocket's outer shell from getting too soggy as it defrosts.

This Is What You Put on Your Toast

I Can't Believe It's Not Butter

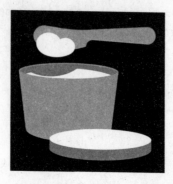

*Start with fat, add more fat, and another fat,
and something that tastes like butter.*

Vegetable Oil Blend (Soybean Oil, Palm Oil, Palm Kernel Oil, Canola Oil)

If I Can't Believe It's Not Butter (henceforth to be known in these pages as ICBINB) is not butter, then what is it? It's not margarine, which by FDA diktat must be at least 80 percent fat. ICBINB is only about 60 percent fat, so it qualifies as a "spread," which is one of those words that seem to have no legal meaning. Since these particular fats are all described as oils (i.e., liquids), how does ICBINB get its semisolid consistency? ICBINB's makers wave away the issue and claim they just add the oils in such a way as to achieve the desired thickness.

Vitamin A Palmitate

Butter abounds with natural vitamin A, something that "spreads" don't come by naturally. Since the FDA demands that all margarine-type foods be "'not nutritionally inferior' to the food that it resembles and for which it substitutes," ICBINB must be fortified. Vitamin A palmitate is simply vitamin A mixed with a bit of palm oil.

Beta-carotene

Beta-carotene is what scientists call a pro-vitamin; that is, it's not a vitamin itself, but the human body converts it to vitamin A, just like the FDA wants. But who doesn't enjoy the thrill of (metaphorically) killing two birds with one stone? Since this molecule is one of the sources of a carrot's orangey color, food chemists also use it to tint ICBINB and other oil spreads a delicate buttery yellow (after all, it would be pretty easy to believe it's not butter if it didn't look anything like butter). It's efficiencies like these that drive the artificial butter market.

Sweet Cream Buttermilk

Still can't believe it's not butter? Take some fresh, "sweet" milk or cream and churn it into real butter. Skim this stuff, which is the leftover liquid, off the top of the butter. Then add it to the vegetable oil spread you want to convince people is butter. This stuff adds a completely natural milky, sweet, buttery flavor to the mix, making even the most die-hard skeptics into true believers.

Soy Lecithin

You know the yellow part of an egg? One of the main chemicals there is called lecithin, which can also come from soy. It contains fats, and it has a yellow color, making it perfect for ICBINB.

Potassium Sorbate

According to the FDA, this additive is generally regarded as safe. According to the USDA, this is the most widely used food preservative in the world and is broken down by the body into nothing more dangerous than potassium, carbon dioxide, and water. Sorbate disrupts the action of at least nine different enzymes used by bacteria and molds, preventing them from breaking down alcohol, generating energy for the cells, digesting carbohydrates, removing ammonia, breaking down hydrogen peroxide, and operating their mitochondria. At that point the microorganisms ask themselves, what's the point of living anymore? Then they die.

Calcium Disodium EDTA

If your name was really ethylenediaminetetraacetic acid, you'd call yourself EDTA, too. The FDA allows it in foodstuffs at anywhere from seventy-five parts per million in margarine to eight hundred parts per million in pinto beans (according to Dow Chemical, which manufactures the stuff, it's also kosher!). While the FDA says that this stuff has many uses, from preservative to color retainer to "anti-gushing agent" in beer, for the most part EDTA is a metal chelator. The multiple oxygen and nitrogen atoms branching off the molecule's core act almost as arms or pincers, encapsulating stray atoms of copper, magnesium, iron, manganese, and calcium that might give the food an off taste or an off color. Poisonous on the cellular level and slightly harmful to mammalian DNA at high doses, EDTA is not thought to be carcinogenic—at least, not as of this writing.

[BACKSTORY]

What is butter? Why is this not butter? Why can't people believe it is not butter?

The FDA is absolutely no help. This is the official government definition of butter, taken from the United States Code (21 USC, chapter 9, subchapter II, sec. 321A):

> For the purposes of the Food and Drug Act of June 30, 1906 (Thirty-fourth Statutes at Large, page 768) "butter" shall be understood to mean the food product usually known as butter, and which is made exclusively from milk or cream, or both, with or without common salt, and with or without additional coloring matter, and containing not less than 80 per centum by weight of milk fat, all tolerances having been allowed for.

Did everyone get that? Butter is defined as being "butter." If you need further definition, you're just a troublemaker. (Incidentally, if you're one of those people who think that the

---

FATTY ACID

A fatty acid is a substance made of an "acid" group (consisting of a carbon atom, two oxygen atoms, and a hydrogen atom, in the configuration -COOH), connected to a hydrocarbon chain (in which carbon atoms are connected in a more or less straight line, with hydrogen atoms branching off from them). When three or more fatty acids are gathered together in the presence of a molecule of glycerol, they generally all join up to make a triglyceride—what we commonly refer to as *fat*. Depending on the length of the fatty acid chains, these substances can be solid or liquid at room temperature. The chains are longer if the substance is liquid; we generally refer to this as oil.

world was simpler years ago, I should point out that that definition was enacted March 4, 1923, nearly one hundred years ago.)

So if butter is defined by the Ayn Randian "A = A," what is margarine? Things are a little clearer here:

> Margarine (or oleomargarine) is the food in plastic form or liquid emulsion, containing not less than 80 percent . . . edible fats and/or oils, or mixtures of these, whose origin is vegetable or rendered animal carcass fats, or any form of oil from a marine species that has been affirmed as a food additive for this use.

But not much. In short, it looks as though butter is a spreadable semisolid substance made from 80 percent milk fat, and margarine is a spreadable semisolid substance made from 80 percent some other kind of fat.

Since these particular fats are all described as oils (i.e., liquids), how does ICBINB get its semisolid consistency? In the old days they hydrogenated the oils. By bubbling H_2 through liquid fats in the presence of a nickel catalyst, scientists add more hydrogen to the fat, changing oil from a liquid to a solid. This process had the unwelcome side effect of sometimes producing trans fats, which are bad for you.

So what is a vegetable oil spread? That doesn't seem to have an FDA definition. By examining ICBINB, we can guesstimate that a spread is a collection of semisolid oils that doesn't meet the 80 percent fat threshold of margarine. At least that's something to believe.

FreshBurst Listerine

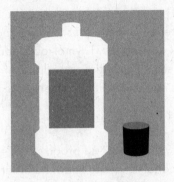

Freshens breath, kills germs, and poisons winos.

Eucalyptol

A spicy, oily extract of the eucalyptus tree, this works almost as well as the steroid prednisone to relax the mucus-producing cells called monocytes in your airways. Most often sniffed or ingested, eucalyptol can be taken in suppository form as an asthma treatment. Suddenly, using an inhaler seems not so bad.

Menthol

The sensors in your body that detect cold are fooled as easily as a tourist in Times Square, and this oily mint derivative is the three-card monte dealer. When ingested or rubbed on the skin, menthol tricks the cold sensors into telling the brain, "We're cool!" thus providing the *sensation* of a thrilling chill without actually cooling your skin. And psychologically, cool equals clean.

Methyl Salicylate

The chief constituent of wintergreen oil, this flavoring—a phenol—is found in root beer, Bengay, and cigarettes. It can also relieve mild aches and pains just like its salicylate cousin aspirin.

Thymol

Like the three previous ingredients, this plant extract is a member of the phenol family, the Genghis Khans of the bacterial world. They kill germs by pillaging the lipids from the inner and outer cell membranes, causing the bacteria's cytoplasm to leak out and die. Thymol, obtained from thyme or oregano, is so strong an antimicrobial that ancient Egyptians (and Evita's embalmers) used it to preserve the dead.

Alcohol

FreshBurst Listerine is almost 44 proof, stronger than a shot of Kahlúa. The alcohol is here to keep the other ingredients dissolved, and it specifically helps to penetrate oral plaque. To keep Listerine from being taxed as liquor, Johnson & Johnson denatures it—making it unpalatable. The company won't give its recipe, but perhaps coincidentally, the US government's Alcohol and Tobacco Tax and Trade Bureau's denaturant formula 38-B contains eucalyptol, menthol, methyl salicylate, and thymol. The chemicals are coming from inside the house!

Sorbitol Solution

The original formulation of Listerine prided itself on its awful taste; now there are yummier alternatives. Sugar promotes cavities, so J & J uses this sweetener that cannot be easily metabolized by normal bacteria. But there's a catch: eating too much sorbitol changes the whole chemical environment of your mouth, which can lead to an increase in the evolution of sorbitol-adapted bacteria in your dental plaque. Nice going, Darwin.

Poloxamer 407

This petroleum-based detergent keeps oily ingredients in solution. Its secret talent is to remain liquid at room temperature but gel at body temp. That weird feeling on your tongue after you gargle could be P407.

. . . .

Benzoic Acid

An aromatic carboxylic acid, this was discovered in 1556 by Nostradamus, of all people, during his alchemy experiments. He could never have predicted it would be used to keep bacteria and mold from growing in mouthwash.

. . . .

FD&C Green #3

The color of a substance depends on the wavelengths of light it reflects and absorbs, and for an organic dye, that depends on the number and type of bonds between its atoms. This particular dye absorbs at 625 nanometers—perfect for displaying blue-green.

. . . .

[BACKSTORY]

I f I'm lucky, when I'm researching one of these stories I'll have a brain-chemistry moment in which all the pieces appear to come together and make a unified whole. With this one, it came when I discovered the Alcohol and Tobacco Tax and Trade Bureau's list of denaturant formulas. Was it just a coincidence that formula 38-B perfectly matched some of the ingredients in Listerine?

Listerine, and other mouthwashes developed approximately one hundred years ago, were marketed with the claim that they kill the germs that cause bad breath. And to this day, there are few substances better at killing germs, while still remaining relatively nontoxic to humans, than pure alcohol. As public hygiene standards increased (and as the power of advertising made people wary of even their most basic biological processes), what could be better than swishing pure ethanol and a few other ingredients around the mouth to kill germs?

Telling people they're not supposed to drink mouthwash is a failure right from the start. As Prohibition showed, people will drink any ethanol-based liquid you hand them. It's why many alcohol rehabs deny this type of mouthwash to their patients. (It's no joke: author Stephen King claimed to be a secret Scope guzzler during his drinking days.)

So the federal government decided to poison the stuff.

Never mind how alcohol itself is a poison; we're talking about adding extra poison in addition to the alcohol that's already in Listerine. The point of these chemicals is to "denature" the alcohol, make you sick to your stomach and throw up. The idea is that you'll never be able to drink enough Listerine to get drunk on without throwing it all up first.

Of course, I had to try this.

I took a deep breath, went into the bathroom, and grabbed the bottle of FreshBurst Listerine. I poured myself one capful, about the size of a large shot glass.

I swallowed it down. I really don't drink, and swallowing any alcohol always comes as a shock to me. I realized, too late, that I had a very good chance not only of getting physically sick from the denaturants but also of getting drunk from a single shot of Listerine.

The first thing I felt was a burning sensation in my chest,

ALCOHOL

Why does our society deem it necessary to place any sort of tax or restriction on the sale of alcohol? No one disagrees that alcohol, consumed irresponsibly, can devastate people, families, and communities. And no responsible adult wants to see alcohol in the hands of children. But few doctors will dispute that alcohol taken responsibly in small amounts can actually be beneficial to one's health. The question then becomes: do the societal benefits of alcohol outweigh the societal damages of alcohol?

A lawyer and lobbyist named Wayne Bidwell Wheeler answered emphatically no! In the late 1880s, he joined the antialcohol temperance movement. Through his phenomenal people skills, along with a developed talent for political arm twisting, Wheeler was the person most responsible for the passage of the Eighteenth Amendment to the US Constitution, which prohibited the manufacture, sale, and import of liquor in the United States.

As a concept, Prohibition might have been a noble experiment. In practice, it resulted in the growth of organized crime, and it fostered a general disrespect for the law, as it turned a nation of social drinkers into criminals.

By 1933, Americans had decided that complete Prohibition was a failure but that some regulation of alcohol was probably a good thing. But the prohibitionists weren't completely powerless. They saw to it that with the repeal of the Eighteenth Amendment came a host of new laws: all drinkable liquor had to have a federal tax stamp, and ethanol not intended for drinking had to be rendered undrinkable by the addition of adulterants. These poisons explain how Listerine gets away with selling ethyl alcohol with a few minty flavorings.

This leads to one unanswerable chicken-or-egg question: did the Listerine people choose their denaturants to fit formula 38-B, or was formula 38-B accepted in order to work with the Listerine people?

exactly the way the American Heart Association describes the early symptoms of a heart attack. The mouthwash burn spread throughout my torso. Was it really possible that I could take a single shot of alcohol and poison and initiate a heart attack? Cardiac problems certainly run in my family, triggered by the most mundane things; my father once had a heart attack while watching PBS. With a genetic legacy like that, I knew that anything was possible.

The warmth—no, the incredible painful burning—settled in my stomach. I nearly doubled over. Then I actually doubled over. Weird drunk thoughts perfused my brain: Would this pain be there forever? Would I, for the rest of my life, be hunched over? Doubled up? Held to ridicule as a casualty of journalism? These are the things you think about when you've drunk Listerine at one a.m.

My stomach slowly accommodated itself to the Listerine. I felt nauseous and sweaty, but there's a difference between "I think I might throw up" and "I'm definitely about to throw up." I was still in the thinking stage, nowhere near the certainty stage. Since I didn't want my last thoughts to be about mouthwash deaths or formula 38-B, I went into the living room and read a book until little bits of daylight showed through the window, when I realized that the pain had subsided and I was still alive.

Midol

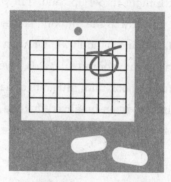

Are you there, God? It's me, nasal decongestant,
wood pulp, and white pigment.

Acetaminophen

This is a key ingredient in many headache remedies, used here
to combat period pains. A one-thousand-milligram dose takes
some of the hex off menstrual cramps (which is a gentle term
for uterine contractions that can be insanely intense), which are
caused by increased prostaglandins and other lipid compounds
in the muscles. Acetaminophen is believed to reduce pain by
activating the brain's CB1 cannabinoid receptors, in effect telling
those prostaglandins to mellow out, dude.

Pyrilamine Maleate

Bayer says this H1 antihistamine is officially here to temporarily
relieve the swelling caused by water retention. Studies have
shown that certain H1 antihistamines can also reduce the total
volume of menstrual loss (e.g., blood and clumps), which has
got to be a good thing. The FDA hasn't given approval for using
antihistamines that way, though, so for now it's all aspirational.

Gelatin—in Midol gelcaps only

Five hundred milligrams of acetaminophen makes for a good-sized tablet, which can be hard to swallow. Pill makers have long coated their offerings in gelatin, which can act like a lubricant when hydrated by saliva, allowing the tablet to slide down the esophagus. One problem: as the gelatin hydrates, it might form a gel layer around the tablet, which keeps it from breaking up and releasing the active ingredients.

Caffeine

Muscle pain can cause increased fatigue: it's exhausting to be in agony. The sixty milligrams of caffeine in each pill can counteract that tiredness; plus, as a diuretic it can relieve menstrual bloat. There's evidence that serious caffeinators (three or more coffees per day) are only a third as likely to menstruate for longer than a week. Midol lattes, anyone?

Lecithin—in Midol gelcaps only

Pill makers use this as an emulsifier and surfactant; it's added to the mix to improve the eventual wetting and dissolution of the active ingredients across the gastrointestinal membrane.

Hypromellose

To the chemist, it's hydroxypropylmethylcellulose. To the layman, it's chemically treated wood pulp and cotton fibers. Here, it's a water-soluble polymer used as a coating and binder in tablets.

Propylene Glycol

This is probably a plasticizer in the tablet coating. The polymer chains of pharmaceutical coatings (even gelatin) might be too brittle to shape themselves around the curves of a tablet. Propylene glycol gets between the polymers, acting like a joint or hinge to give them the elasticity to bend when necessary.

Croscarmellose Sodium

This superdisintegrant causes the pill to blow apart in your stomach, making it much more fast acting.

Titanium Dioxide

A white pigment that may also act as a shield. Drug molecules can be fragile things—acetaminophen and caffeine are broken down by light, which eventually makes them useless. This opacifier can reflect visible rays, keeping the inside of the pill in the dark.

Triacetin

Remember when we thought astronauts were going to have to synthesize their own food on long space voyages (remember when we thought astronauts were going to *have* long space voyages)? In at least one NASA plan, their interplanetary menu was going to be based around this stuff, an easily metabolized water-soluble triglyceride. Here on Earth, it is added to butter to help enhance the flavor; it is also sometimes used as an antifungal agent and as a rocket fuel component (don't ask). Pharmaceutically, it is used here as a solvent for the active ingredients as a way to achieve a uniform distribution.

Black Iron Oxide

The ink used to print "Midol" on the side of the tablet. Just so you know who's making you feel less awful.

Simethicone—in Midol gelcaps only

A key ingredient in antiburp products like Gas-X, this silicone polymer lowers the surface tension of little gas bubbles, causing them to gather together into one giant bubble that is more easily passed. Here it is used to make sure that the lecithin doesn't foam up in the factory. Also can be added to the gel coating to prevent unsightly air bubbles.

Shellac

The same smelly stuff your dad coated the deck with during the Carter administration? Yes; at least this stuff is pharmaceutical grade. A sticky excretion of Southeast Asian lac insects, it could be an ingredient in the ink, or it might be here to provide a natural hard coating on the tablet.

. . . .

MENSTRUAL RELIEF

Nearly four thousand years ago, ancient Egyptians treated their menstrual symptoms with a poultice made of wood pulp! Of course, their medicine also included things like the smoke from the thighs of orioles and fresh donkey liver.

Okay, to put it bluntly the Egyptian pharmacopoeia was essentially useless for relieving menstrual pain. But it shows the lengths to which women would go to get some temporary relief every month (and it also gives an insight into the absolute fascination that some men—from pharaonic doctors to Republican senators—have with the female reproductive system). The simple fact is that throughout history, the only menstrual relief that has ever worked has been standard pain relief things: exercise and plant-based teas and extracts. (Stuffy old Queen Victoria was a monthly stoner, regularly taking a liquid extract of *Cannabis indica* [i.e., medical marijuana] for her menstrual cramps.)

In the laissez-faire days before there were any sort of food or drug regulations, shady entrepreneurs sold substances called "patent medicines," which were usually touted as being able to cure menstrual discomfort and just about anything else that ailed you. What they really cured was the *pain* of just about anything, because patent medicines were essentially nothing more than laudanum: opium dissolved in alcohol, delivering two addictions for the price of one. As more and more women turned to these laudanum products for relief, they found themselves hooked. Medical historians estimate that there were between 150,000 and 200,000 opiate addicts in the United States in the late 1880s, and about 75 percent of them were women.

Orbit White Gum

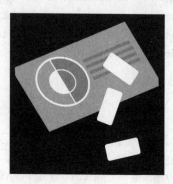

Fake sugar, boiled pine, and NASCAR tires.

Maltitol

This is one of a family of mild sweeteners known as sugar alcohols, or polyols. Typically derived from natural carbs, they lack the harsh, metallic taste of most calorie-free sweeteners. Sugar alcohols are absorbed very slowly (or not at all) in the intestines, so they don't cause spikes in blood-sugar level (not that diabetics should go nuts with the stuff). And since oral bacteria can't digest them, they won't rot your teeth. Why isn't everything sweetened this way? Well, for one thing, that slow intestinal absorption can cause bloating, diarrhea, and flatulence.

. . . .

Sorbitol

More sugar alcohol. Here, a simple glucose molecule ($C_6H_{12}O_6$) is broken apart and two extra hydrogen atoms are added (making $C_6H_{14}O_6$). The result is about half as sweet as the original molecule. But while it sounds like a Frankensteinian laboratory monstrosity, it's not; sorbitol can also be found naturally in peaches, plums, and other fruit.

. . . .

Gum Base

Chewing gum used to be made from the sap of manilkara trees, but now the chew often comes from styrene-butadiene, the same petrochemical rubber used to make automobile tires. Wrigley won't divulge its recipe but claims to still use some natural ingredients in its gum base—like, oh, boiled pine sap.

Glycerol

The sugar alcohols just keep on coming. This clear, syrupy liquid, also known as glycerin, is a favorite in pharmaceuticals and personal care products for its smooth texture and moisturizing properties. A by-product of biodiesel production, glycerol is now flooding global markets as more life-based fuel is manufactured. Plans are afoot to turn it into eco-friendly antifreeze.

Aspartame

This stuff was being used in the development of an anti-ulcer drug in 1965 when a researcher for pharmaceutical giant Searle absentmindedly licked his fingers. After he was no doubt reprimanded for poor laboratory discipline, he realized that this stuff was about two hundred times more sweetly potent than sugar. Here, the calorie-free additive compensates for the modest sweetness of sugar alcohols with a big blast of cloy. A synthesis of two naturally occurring amino acids, it breaks down into small amounts of toxic chemicals like methanol and formaldehyde in the body. What's the problem? The FDA isn't worried, so why should you be?

Acesulfame K

Is this some geeky hip-hop name? No, the "K" stands for potassium. This is another cloyingly intense calorie-free sweetener. It's rarely used alone, since it packs a particularly bitter aftertaste. Unlike aspartame, ace K is totally artificial, so the body doesn't even try to metabolize it—in layman's terms, you just piss it away.

. . . .

Sodium Bicarbonate

Orbit White's unique selling point is that it's supposed to help whiten your unsightly chompers. Enter sodium bicarbonate—good old baking soda—a plaque inhibitor and gentle abrasive that cleans teeth without damaging the enamel. Boo-yah! We can finally stop brushing our teeth.

. . . .

[BACKSTORY]

In one of his greatest articles ("The Last American Hero Is Junior Johnson. Yes!"), the writer Tom Wolfe described, among other things, the origins of NASCAR racing. Wolfe explained how, during the early test or qualifying runs in the NASCAR circuit, the pit crew will put very soft rubber tires on the car. These tires hold tight on the corners, which is what you need for qualifying, and were colloquially known as "gumballs." These gumball tires tended to smoke and deteriorate pretty rapidly, leaving a circle of gray-blue haze in the sky over the track. In Wolfe's words, this would prompt the locals to shout, "GREAT SMOKIN BLUE GUMBALLS GOD ALMIGHTY DOG!"

It's quite possible that one reason those tires are called gumballs is because in fact those tires are made of the same type of rubber used in chewing gum. That's right: styrene-butadiene is the rubber that is the basis of your chewing gum.

Don't get too disgusted by this revelation. Rubber is essentially the thickened sap of a tropical latex tree. Chicle, the original source of chewing gum and the origin of the word "Chiclets," is the thickened sap from a slightly different tropical tree. They're both very similar in structure and composition. Whether you're chewing original chicle gum or more modern synthetic latex gum, you're basically masticating pretty much the same molecules over and over and over and over again. However, just knowing that sometimes isn't enough.

Once, when my girlfriend Emily and I were at the supermarket, we were just getting on the checkout line when she looked at our full cart and said, "You forgot your gum." I was silent. She knew that every time we went food shopping, we always got a giant package of chewing gum for me. And we didn't get it this time. I didn't say a word, but Emily is no dummy. She said, "What are you working on right now?" I couldn't hold it back any longer. "I'm researching the chemistry of chewing gum!" I said with an exaggerated sob. She said, "You're doing chewing gum and suddenly you've *stopped* chewing gum?" I could only nod. She said, "I do *not* want to know what you found." I said, "A lot of people agree with you."

PowerBar ProteinPlus

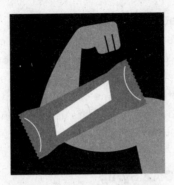

In which we finally learn the difference between chocolate and chocolatey.

Whey Protein Isolate

These are globular proteins (of the same general structure as hemoglobin in the blood and gamma globulin in the immune system) left over from cheese-making, minus the fats and sugars. The main protein, beta-lactoglobulin, is interesting: it has no known biological function other than to serve as an especially good source of amino acids for building other proteins.

Calcium Caseinate

Another milk-derived protein, more slowly digested than whey protein isolate. Legend had it that casein could worsen autism due to the protein's alleged opiate-like effects on the brain. But a 2006 study showed no significant connection. So don't blame PowerBar for your Asperger's, nerdlinger.

Soy Protein Isolate

Protein extracted from ground-up soybeans, with the fats and sugars removed. High intake of soy protein has been linked to lower rates of coronary heart disease. But manly men seeking to

develop Schwarzeneggerian musculature may not like the fact
that it's rich in phytoestrogens (plant-based girlie hormones).

Chocolatey Coating

What's the difference between chocolate and chocolatey?
Anything sold as "chocolate" can contain only one type of added
fat—cocoa butter. But add a "-y," and you can sell cocoa mixed
with lard or any other fat, none of which have the heart-friendly
effects of cocoa butter. PowerBars use fractionated palm kernel
oil instead, which is about as healthy as Elmer's Glue-All.

High-Fructose Corn Syrup

This ingredient is everywhere, even in so-called health foods. In
2006, Americans consumed fifty-eight pounds of this sweetener
per capita, up nearly fifty pounds in thirty years.

Glycerin

The bar's chewy texture is due in part to this sugar alcohol,
which moonlights as a food moisturizer.

Maltitol Syrup

A twelve-carbon sugar alcohol and probable sweetener, but
one that the body absorbs super slowly. Besides gas and
bloating, maltitol can produce a laxative effect so powerful
that Australia and New Zealand require a warning label on
foods that contain it.

Oat Fiber

Oat fiber helps lower cholesterol by fermenting into the short-
chain fatty acid butyrate, which can limit the release of lipids
from the small intestine. At last, eight ingredients in, something
truly healthy in a health bar!

Calcium Phosphate

This supposed performance enhancer (which is essentially powdered bonelike minerals) is also used to polish teeth and build hard-tissue prosthetics.

Copper Gluconate

In theory, a copper deficiency can lead to anemia and neurological disorders (though such problems are usually found only in people who have been kept alive via intravenous feeding or in babies fed nothing but cow's milk). So copper gluconate sounds healthy. Too bad a 1985 study showed zero effects from adding it to the diet.

Pantothenic Acid (Calcium Pantothenate)

Better known as vitamin B5, pantothenic acid is necessary for the digestion of sugars, proteins, and fats. Handily, it's found widely in foods—plants, animals, and all PowerBar ProteinPluses.

Vitamin B6

B6 is essential for the synthesis of neurotransmitters like epinephrine, norepinephrine, dopamine, and serotonin. But don't binge, new moms: too much can stop lactation.

FAT FREE, NONFAT, LOW FAT, LIGHT

Only in the bizarro world of food labeling can the terms "fat free," "zero fat," "no fat," and "without fat" not necessarily mean that the product in fact has zero grams of fat. In the world according to the FDA, "zero" means anything from actually zero all the way up to half a gram. By this outlandish arithmetic, four servings of "zero fat" food can actually contain close to two grams of fat.

The situation is caused by two diametrically opposed camps with differing needs. The American public has been rendered fearful of fatty food (while simultaneously loving fatty food). They've taken it to heart that a reduction in consumed fat is automatically good for them.

At the same time, food manufacturers are deeply in love with fat. Fat is relatively inexpensive! Fat makes food taste great! Fat gives food an unbeatably seductive mouthfeel. Fat can literally be as addictive as cocaine and heroin. Fat keeps 'em coming back for more!

So, torn between these two forces, the FDA has to make compromises that, ultimately, make no sense. For example, "low fat" means that the food in question contains less than three grams of fat per serving. Unless the food in question is milk. Milk is special; low-fat milk gets to have up to five grams of fat per serving, because the low-fat guidelines for milk were established in the 1970s and get to be grandfathered in.

"Light" means that the food gets less than 50 percent of its calories from fat. If you buy a package of cookies that are one hundred calories per serving, and forty-nine of those calories come from fat, that is officially a "light" (also permitted: "lite") cookie.

"Light" (or "lite") can also mean that the caloric count of the product has been artificially reduced by one-third compared to the original version of the food. So imagine this scenario: You have a product that's normally one hundred fifty calories per serving, with forty-nine calories (about one-third) coming from fat. Your food scientists go to work and produce a version of the product that has only one hundred calories per serving, with the same forty-nine calories (about one-half) coming from fat. In what is probably the most insane FDA rule ever, that new formulation is officially a "lite" product, even though the percentage of calories from fat has risen.

Red Bull

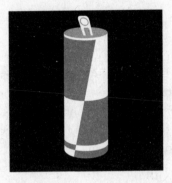

Wings? This doesn't even give you feathers.

Glucose

Like most popular soft drinks, Red Bull is largely sugar water. But don't count on its glucose to "give you wings," as the ad says. Multiple studies have debunked the so-called sugar high.

Taurine

Also known as 2-aminoethanesulfonic acid, taurine was originally isolated from bull bile in 1827. Now made synthetically, it is the magical elixir said to bring out the kite-surfing extremophile in any web-surfing nerd. Taurine's actual effects, while not as drastic as the hype, are pretty wide-ranging, even from the amount found in a single can of Red Bull: not only is it an inhibitory neurotransmitter (in some cases acting as a mild sedative) and an age-defying antioxidant, it even has the potential to steady irregular heartbeats.

Glucuronolactone

Internet rumors claimed this was a Vietnam-era experimental drug that caused brain tumors. Luckily, that's not true. But don't crumple up your tinfoil hat yet—hardly anyone has looked into exactly what this stuff does. So little research has been done on glucuronolactone (and most of it fifty years ago) that almost all information about it is mere rumor. Users generally believe it fights fatigue and increases well-being, but that could turn out to be bull, too.

. . . .

Caffeine
Ah, *here* are Red Bull's wings. All the things this drink is supposed to do for you—increase concentration and reaction speed, improve emotional state, and boost metabolism—are known effects of this white powder, a distant cousin of cocaine. Unfortunately, too much caffeine can also lead to irregular heartbeat, jitteriness, and frequent urination—soooooo uncool when you're trying to make a good impression. Good thing there's taurine to smooth out those arrhythmias.

. . . .

Niacin (Niacinamide)
Also known as vitamin B3, niacin increases so-called good cholesterol (HDL) by preventing the formation of triglycerides, making it a terrific cholesterol drug. Unfortunately, there isn't enough niacin here to have this benefit. And it's not even pure enough to give you the mild head rush dubbed the "niacin flush."

. . . .

Sodium Citrate
Commonly used as a preservative in soft drinks and spreadable cheeses, sodium citrate also helps convert glucose into lactic acid during exercise, producing a measurable effect on athletic performance. In at least one test, it shaved an average of seventeen seconds off a 5K run. Unfortunately, it's also a laxative, so watch where you step.

. . . .

Inositol
A carbohydrate found in many places, but most surprisingly in animal muscle (where it is sometimes called "meat sugar"), inositol is turning out to be a wonder drug. Studies have

shown that it significantly reduces depression, panic attacks, agoraphobia, and obsessive-compulsive disorder. It might even be what makes whole grains effective cancer fighters. Instead of being a bit player in Red Bull (you'd need to drink as many as 360 cans a day to get its benefits), inositol probably deserves a drink of its own.

. . . .

ANTIOXIDANT

Much of the body's life processes are a carefully balanced collection of oxidation and reduction reactions. On occasion, these reactions get out of balance, either caused by or resulting in a free radical, a molecule with unpaired electrons. These free radicals can start oxidative chain reactions; they can create new free radicals by stealing electrons from normal molecules. These new free radicals then go on to damage more molecules, which then go on to do even more damage. An antioxidant puts a stop to the carnage by providing the free radical with electrons without itself becoming a free radical.

This Is What You Put in Your Glass

Red Wine

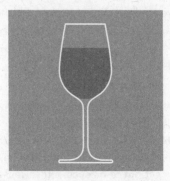

In vino veritas, along with antioxidants, sour milk juice, and a migraine trigger.

Ethanol

Nearly every culture on Earth sees something magical, even holy, about the fact that microorganisms eat sugar ($C_6H_{12}O_6$), rearrange the atoms, and excrete this toxin (CH_3CH_2O), which we then drink to confuse the smart parts of our brain into thinking that we are gods.

. . . .

Glycerol

This is a syrupy sugar alcohol, a by-product of ethanol fermentation. Oenophiles will lecture you for hours about how glycerol influences a wine's "body" and "silkiness." But does it? Despite the claim of some winemakers that it is as important to a wine's mouthfeel as ethanol, chemists know that the fraction of glycerol in wine has little detectable impact on the viscosity. They suggest looking to yeast cell wall proteins and phenol compounds instead.

. . . .

Tannins

These bitter, astringent molecules found in dark grape skins (and in the oak barrels used to age fine wine) do a real number on your tongue. Their multiple phenol groups bind to salivary proteins, making your mouth feel drier than it should feel when it's full of liquid. This odd effect is what oenophiles call a "gripping" mouthfeel.

Malvidin 3-Glucoside

One of a family of natural pigments called anthocyanins, also found in cranberries and blueberries. Also known as oenin, it puts the red in red wine.

Catechin and Caffeic Acid

Catechin is a phenol antioxidant found in grape seeds. Caffeic acid is another phenolic compound found in grapes. Together they have the serendipitous benefit of preventing bodily damage from ionizing radiation: catechin keeps chromosomes safe, while caffeic acid fights radiation damage by wandering the body neutralizing any reactive oxygen molecules that have been let loose by stray gamma rays. Send a magnum to your local nuclear plant workers for when they're off duty.

3-Isobutyl-2-Methoxy-Pyrazine

This chemical (a.k.a. IBMP) gives Cabernet Sauvignon its herbaceous green pepper aroma, detectable at as little as six parts per trillion. Connoisseurs note: if the smell is overpowering, it could mean the grapes were not allowed sufficient time to ripen—IBMP breaks down as grapes mature. Or leaves may have gotten into the ferment (the green parts of the vine are chock-full of IBMP).

Tyramine

Wine-and-cheese parties give you a migraine? It might not be the pretentious banter. You could be overdosing on this amino acid, which is found in both of these edibles. Tyramine constricts cerebral blood vessels; when it wears off, the blood vessels dilate on the rebound, which causes a throbbing headache. So skip the cheese, but be sure to nosh on something; you'll absorb less tyramine if you have food in your stomach.

Malic and Lactic Acids

Malic acid occurs naturally in grapes. But too much of it gives vino a harsh "green" taste that clashes with other flavors. Most vintners let the wine age a bit so bacteria can turn malic acid into the "softer," "rounder" lactic acid. But it's a tricky business: too much lactic acid can give wine a sauerkraut flavor.

Resveratrol

The antioxidant that's been touted for the past decade as red wine's miracle cure-all: It fights cancer! It tames diabetes! It keeps winos alive forever! But it is also the real reason Dracula never drinks wine: resveratrol and other polyphenols inhibit the stomach's absorption of dietary iron; in the lab, regular use can bring on anemia among susceptible mice. And anemia is the last thing Dracula needs.

[BACKSTORY]

Wine has so many fantastic ingredients—we counted at least seventy specific ingredients, in fourteen major molecular groups—that we had a hard time culling it to "only" eleven. We tried to include one ingredient from each group but literally ran out of space.

Unlike the other commodities I have analyzed, like coffee, cigarettes, or gasoline, there has never been any serious legal investigation into the ingredients of red wine. When I looked at the ingredients of cigarettes I was helped immensely by the findings of the various tobacco lawsuits of the 1990s.

ACID

One of the first things you learn about in grade school science class is that vinegar is an acid and it can make baking soda fizzle into foam. But what *is* an acid, really? There are three different definitions: According to the Swedish chemist Svante Arrhenius (1859-1927), an acid is any substance that produces hydrogen ions (H+) or hydronium (H_3O) when dissolved in water. According to Danish chemist Johannes Nicolaus Brønsted (1879-1947) and English chemist Thomas Martin Lowry (1874-1936), who each arrived at the theory independently, an acid is any substance that can donate a proton in a chemical reaction, while a base can accept a proton. The American chemist Gilbert Newton Lewis (1875-1946) defined an acid as any substance that can accept an electron pair from another atom to complete one of its own atoms. It all seems pretty complicated, but the bottom line is that an acid is a substance that can't help but react with certain other substances, either by donating a proton or accepting electrons. In many of our products, acids provide a tangy or sour taste—that is the effect of hydrogen ions on the taste buds.

Gasoline, being a known health hazard, has also been seriously investigated. But there's very little useful information on the actual chemical components of red wine. Many of the professional vintners I've spoken to claim not to even know the various chemicals inside their wines. Whether they're telling the truth or whether they just don't want to talk about it, the result is that it's extremely difficult to learn about wine on a molecular level.

The best peer-reviewed resources available are the various studies that have been done on the health properties of red wine. But these usually focus on the compound resveratrol, which, as we have seen, is touted as everything from a cure for cancer to a fountain of youth.

Curiously enough, some of the most interesting information about wine comes not from professional wineries but from home winemakers. These are folks just like you or me, trying to do something cool at home by turning grapes into wine. As such they have the keen specialized knowledge of the enthusiast. Many of them claim not to have known any chemistry at all before they got involved in winemaking. Now they can talk about tannins and esters along with Ph.D. chemists.

I know everyone's question is going to be: how many bottles of wine did you drink to write this particular chapter? Sorry to disappoint but the answer is none. It was all done from research.

Samuel Adams Harvest Pumpkin Ale

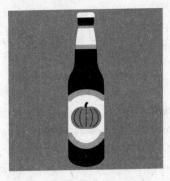

Yeasty Halloween goodness from the father of the American Revolution, or something like that.

Two-Row Barley

About eight thousand years ago, "normal" barley, which has two rows of grains per stalk, mutated to become six-row barley. Mesolithic humans were probably thrilled with the increased yield, but like all mutants, the new barley came to be hated and feared by at least one segment of the population. Beer makers soon realized that six-row barley has less flavor and starch compared to two-row barley, making it less than ideal for brewing a batch. (To this day, American brewers tend to use six-row barley, but in Europe it's pretty much exclusively two-row.)

Caramel 60 and Smoked Malt

The barley is then malted—that is, it is steeped in warm water to germinate it (length of time and temperature of water is a trade secret), which tricks the grain into thinking that it's been planted. At that point, the grain releases enzymes that break its stored stable starch molecules into simple sugars to feed the sprout, on its way to becoming a majestic barley plant. But the joke's on the sprout: at this point, the brewers dry the grain to stop the process! Barley that's destined to become Caramel

60 is roasted to give it caramel notes; the other malt is smoked over a mixed alder-wood and beech-wood fire (reminiscent of bacon!). The result is specialized malted barley, ready for the brewery. Why the different processes? Each bottle of ale contains about three ounces of malt; some double bocks contain a half pound—comparable to a loaf of bread!

Hops

The principal spice in beer. Hops are the female flowers of the plant *Humulus lupulus,* which is also the Hogwarts spell for making ale. You thought barley was temperamental? Hops have all the same terroir issues of wine grapes: soil, climate, region, etc. all combine to make each batch of hops unique. Hops have a natural bacteriostatic quality that inhibits the growth of bacteria that can spoil the flavor of beer, so they (along with the alcohol) are a natural preservative for beer. And they taste good. This beer uses a blend of two varieties of hops: East Kent Goldings, grown in the heart of English hop country for centuries, and an earthy cultivar called (of all things) Fuggles.

Pumpkin

Here to add some sugar and flavor. Like the barley itself, some parts of the pumpkin (for example, the fibers) get filtered out of the final beer. The part of the pumpkin that remains comes to roughly one ounce of pumpkin per bottle. Pumpkin (like malt) also contributes to the mouthfeel of the ale; the fleshy fruit gives the drink a silkier texture.

Top-Fermenting Ale Yeast

Any good brewer will tell you that they don't make beer. They make carefully designed and calibrated yeast food, and the yeast makes the beer by turning that food into alcohol and carbon dioxide. Actually, it's a lot more complicated than that: these little *Saccharomyces cerevisiae* fungi also produce hundreds of rougher, fruitier flavor elements that provide a big part of the aleness of ale. "Top-fermenting" is actually a misnomer: ale yeast ferments quickly, in the space of a week or two, everywhere throughout the beer, and then floats to the top of the vat, where it can be skimmed off (lager yeast, in contrast, tends to take about a month to ferment, before sinking to the bottom of the vat).

Clove

That unique clove smell you find in over-the-counter toothache remedies and obnoxious hipster cigarettes? That's eugenol, a phenol-related compound that is used as a chemical warfare agent. Used by plants, that is, against creatures like us. As players in the "eat or be eaten" world of nature, plants have an enormous strategic deficiency—they can't retreat when they are attacked. Instead, they've evolved to protect themselves by using noxious chemicals to keep vermin and other predators away. But what would be a sickening dose of eugenol for a little critter is nothing but a piquant spice for large animals like humans. And, in a bizarre twist, this actually may have helped the plants—we've become so addicted to spice that we protect and nurture the plants and spread their genes all around the planet. You can't ask for better symbiotic behavior than that.

Cinnamon

It's quite possible that you've never had "true" cinnamon, which is made from the bark of Sri Lankan trees. Much of what is sold as cinnamon in the western world is really cassia, a tree bark with a stronger oil and more bite; true cinnamon is mild, delicate, and sweet, while cassia is more pungent and peppery. It's mildly toxic; ingestion of enough of one of the component chemicals (called coumarin) of cassia cinnamon can lead to liver damage. The best cinnamon? According to a blind taste test Samuel Adams did, the most aromatic, flavorful, and complex cinnamon comes from Vietnam, specifically from the area around Saigon.

. . . .

Ginger

Another plant-based WMD. Remember how Grandma used to give you dry toast and ginger ale when you had a stomach bug? Granny was right; zingerone, the main chemical responsible for ginger's bite, is toxic toward diarrhea-producing *E. coli* bacteria.

. . . .

Allspice

This descendant of the myrtle family is one of the few spices native to the Western Hemisphere, specifically the Caribbean (Jamaica seems to control the allspice industry as a dominant producer) and Central America. Its giant trees, stretching some fifty feet tall, produce berries that, when dried, early European explorers mistook for (or fraudulently claimed were) black peppercorn. When ground, the powder smells like a mixture of cloves, cinnamon, and nutmeg (hence "all spice," duh).

. . . .

[BACKSTORY]

This was one of the most fun pieces to do, because I got to spend an hour with Jim Koch, the cofounder and chairman of the Boston Beer Company, brewers of Samuel Adams. Like all geeks, Jim is insanely enthusiastic when he talks about the thing he loves, which is making beer; he prefaced most of his sentences with "I'll just give you probably more information than you really wanted," which proved he didn't know us very well.

And boy howdy did he deliver. If you're not a farmer or a brewer, you probably think barley is barley is barley, right? Well, apparently there are at least 24 different strains of barley grown in the United States alone; Great Britain grows 146, Germany 120. And each of these barley strains, as we've seen, gives a distinct personality to the beer it makes. Just as there are "good years" for specific wine grapes, there are good and bad years for barley and hops, depending on the weather; the 2013 drought in the Midwest really hurt barley yields.

Koch also elaborated on double bocks: if beer is fattening enough, why would anyone make a beer that's the equivalent of a loaf of bread? According to Koch, "Double bock is a style of beer invented by monks during the Middle Ages to get them through Lent." The rule was that the monks had to fast during Lent, but the loophole was that they still could drink. And did they ever. According to Koch, by overloading beer with barley, the monks could live quite well on this very malty, more alcoholic beer. My Sicilian grandfather used to say that a person who bends the rules is "as tricky as a priest"—this kind of behavior is clearly what he meant.

MAILLARD REACTION

Dark beer. Blackened Cajun chicken. Well-done hamburger. These intense flavors and dark earthy colors are caused by a specific set of physiochemical processes called the Maillard reaction, named after Louis Maillard, the French scientist who first explained it. Unlike ordinary caramelization, which is the browning of simple sugars, the Maillard reaction involves the interplay of a sugar, an amino acid, and heat. Five-carbon sugars like fructose work best, followed by glucose and then more complex sugars. Among the amino acids, lysine gives the most browning, cysteine the least. When heat is applied to the sugars and aminos, they combine to form a compound called glycosylamine. As the heat continues, glycosylamine rearranges itself into hundreds of different compounds, based on the elements available in the sugars and aminos. Practically every aroma associated with cooked foods—savory peptides, oniony sulfur compounds, earthy pyrazines, and nutty furans—is made by the Maillard reaction. The end result of this chemical do-si-do are the brown/black-brown nitrogenous polymers and copolymers called melanoidins. The Maillard reaction is so important that the International Maillard Reaction Society was established in 2005, as they put it, "in response to a growing recognition of the role reactive carbonyl compounds play in food technology, nutrition and tissue aging in biology and medicine."

Finally, Koch and I ended up taking a great deal of time to talk about the head on a mug of beer. Beer foam is made of small spheres of carbon dioxide surrounded by a thin protein chain. Outside the bubble is a near CO_2 vacuum, so the bubble expands, the protein chain stretches and snaps, and the bubble pops. On a Samuel Adams, the head is thick enough to float a bottle cap, because the beer is overloaded with malt proteins that keep the bubbles together longer.

One sneaky way to get a longer-lasting head without adding to the proteinaceous richness of the beer is to inject nitrogen gas into the solution. Nitrogen is closer to equilibrium with the atmosphere, so as a result you get a smaller, longer-lasting bubble. You could hear the scorn in Koch's voice when he said, "It has nothing to do with the beer itself, it has to do with the nitrogen injection into the beer!"

"Oh, this is absolutely fascinating," I said in fanboyish rapture.

"Well, beer is its own physics lesson," Koch said.

This Is What You Put in Your Mouth

Slim Jim

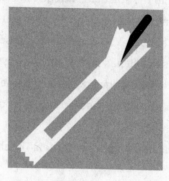

How would you describe your meat stick? Try "alive."

Beef

It's real meat, all right. But it ain't Kobe. The US Department of Agriculture categorizes beef in eight grades of quality. The bottom three grades—Utility, Cutter, and Canner—are typically used in processed foods and come from older steers with partially ossified vertebrae, tougher tissue, and generally less reason to live. ConAgra, whose brands include Banquet, Chef Boyardee, Egg Beaters, Healthy Choice, Hebrew National, Hunt's, Marie Callender's, Odom's Tennessee Pride, Orville Redenbacher's, PAM, Peter Pan, Reddi-wip, and Snack Pack, wasn't exactly forthcoming on what's inside Slim Jims.

Mechanically Separated Chicken

Did you imagine a conveyor belt carrying live chickens into a giant machine, set to the classic cartoon theme "Powerhouse"? You're right! Well, maybe not about the music. Poultry scraps are pressed mechanically through a sieve that extrudes the meat as a bright pink paste and leaves the bones behind—most of the time. Occasionally, there is enough bone residue in just one serving of chicken nuggets to provide up to half the daily allowance of fluoride.

Paprika and Paprika Extractives

Paprika is simply a variety of red bell pepper ground into a fine powder. But what are "extractives"? Because it is listed apart from other spices and flavorings, perhaps the "extractive" is oleoresin of paprika, which gives a meaty red color to sausages and other processed meats.

Corn and Wheat Proteins

Slim Jim is made by ConAgra, which calls itself the "largest private brand food company in America." If there are two things ConAgra has a lot of, it's corn and wheat, along with oats, soybeans, beef, pork, and poultry.

Hydrolyzed Soy

Hydrolysis, in this instance, is the act of using water to break a larger soy protein molecule into its constituent amino acids, such as glutamic acid. One way to do this is to take a quantity of soybeans (usually what remains after the beans have been shucked and oiled) and pressure-cook them in dilute hydrochloric acid. When the resulting soup is neutralized, the end product consists of eighteen different amino acids from soy. Typically, the process also results in glutamic acid salt—also known as monosodium glutamate, a familiar flavor enhancer. What? You didn't see monosodium glutamate on the label? It doesn't have to be listed separately if it comes with the hydrolyzed soy.

Lactic Acid Starter Culture

Although ConAgra refers to Slim Jim as a meat stick (yum), it has a lot in common with old-fashioned fermented sausages like salami and pepperoni. They all use bacteria and sugar to produce lactic acid, which lowers the pH of the sausage to around 5.0, firming up the meat and hopefully killing all harmful bacteria. Even though lactic acid is generally regarded as a milk product, fear not, lactose intolerants: Slim Jim's particular starter culture is safely vegetable based. Not that vegans are going to come anywhere near a Slim Jim.

Dextrose

Serves as food for the lactic acid starter culture. Slim Jim: it's alive!

Salt

In ancient times, people began salting meat to prevent it from spoiling. What happens (though they hardly knew it at the time) is that salt binds the water molecules in meat, leaving little H_2O available for microbial activity—thereby preventing spoilage. This water activity level is crucial: a nonrefrigerated sausage like Slim Jim has to have a water-activity reading of 0.85, about the same as dry cheese. The flip side is that one Slim Jim gives you more than one-sixth of the sodium your body needs in a day.

Sodium Nitrite

Cosmetically, this is added to sausage because it combines with myoglobin in animal muscle to keep it from turning gray. Antibiotically, it inhibits botulism. Toxicologically, six grams of the stuff—roughly the equivalent of fourteen hundred Slim Jims—can kill you. So go easy there, champ.

EXPIRATION DATES

When packaging says "Best if used by [a certain date]" or "Freshest before [a certain date]," it means exactly that: the product is "best" and "freshest" before those dates, and there is a good chance the food will remain adequate, if not so fresh, well after that date. But there is no federal law that says that foods must contain an expiration date, or that foods cannot be sold after the date printed on the packaging. In fact, there is no federal regulation to date food at all; any expiration dates you see on food packaging are there entirely at the discretion of the manufacturer. In certain local jurisdictions, easily perishable products like milk might be packaged with an enforceable sell-by date, but that's done on the state level; the FDA has nothing to do with that.

This Is What You Put in Your Mug

Southern Comfort Egg Nog

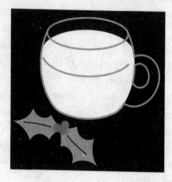

Eggs, milk, spices, and a thirty-year government coverup.

Egg Yolks

Home recipes for eggnog call for six to twelve eggs per quart of milk. This version of eggnog—which usually shows up in grocery stores just in time for the holidays—contains far fewer eggs; based on the total cholesterol content, we estimate that it has just two large egg yolks per quart. Because eggnog contains both dairy and eggs, the FDA has the right to butt in on its contents. But the FDA's requirements are pretty low; the agency expects commercial nog to contain at least 1 percent "egg yolk solids." The math works for us.

Guar Gum

This is the ground-up endosperm of the guar bean. It is used here as a thickener, probably in place of the extra egg yolks we were expecting.

Cream

The FDA also dictates that US nog have at least 6 percent milk fat. Since whole milk is only about 3.5 percent, many manufacturers add a dollop of cream to boost the lipids.

Milk

As we all know, milk can contain entire civilizations of live bacteria that can cause it to spoil quickly. Back in the old days, a bit of alcohol mixed into the milk may have helped kill off some of those bugs. Hundreds of years ago in Britain, milk was sometimes consumed as posset: a potion of milk, eggs, figs, and wine or ale—sound familiar, like some sort of proto-eggnog? Alas, there's no actual Southern Comfort in Southern Comfort Egg Nog, so you will still have to refrigerate this stuff.

Carrageenan

Homemade eggnog (the kind with a dozen cholesterol-laden eggs, remember) has a custardy texture. But ready-made store-bought versions of nog are required to contain just a small percentage of egg solids. So food manufacturers rely on additives like this—a seaweed extract—to thicken their beverage to a familiar consistency.

Corn Syrup

Early Romans had noglike drinks, which they often sweetened with honey. Using corn syrup might be a poor attempt to re-create a thick, homemade texture while simultaneously feeding our sweet tooth. Or it could be a way to save money: real sugar is about 1.4 times more expensive than this stuff.

Spices

Nutmeg is the preferred eggnog seasoning—for many people, the aroma of nutmeg *is* the smell of eggnog. That's probably because back in the days of merrie olde England, nutmeg was costly enough to help make a mug of nog an expensive holiday treat. Nowadays, spices are so readily available that there are commercial eggnog varieties built around nearly every Yuletide spice. (Southern Comfort–branded nog comes in a vanilla-spiked version, and other companies offer pumpkin, caramel, gingerbread, and sugar cookie flavors.) Some reviewers note that Southern Comfort nog has clear clove overtones, with at least a touch of cinnamon.

. . . .

Natural and Artificial Flavor

If the eggnoggy flavor is in the spices, this is likely the "Southern Comfort" taste. According to flavor expert David Dafoe, a whiskey-bourbon taste can be engineered from a mixture of oak extracts (conjuring the oak barrels in which the spirits are aged), a touch of vanilla, and the fruity esters ethyl acetate and ethyl-2-methyl butyrate. How can makers of nonalcoholic beverages like this replicate the "burn" of alcohol on the tongue? Just add a tiny bit of capsicum pepper to the mix. But just enough to bite, not enough to taste!

. . . .

Annatto and Turmeric (for Color)

The use of these two natural food colorings—which add a yellow tone—is technically forbidden in eggnog under federal regulation (it might make revelers think the drink contains more egg than it really does). But eggnog makers pushed back, and that rule has been stayed—pending a public hearing—for the past thirty years! The FDA is now looking into it.

. . . .

[BACKSTORY]

When I decided to look closely at eggnog, as part of the usual research I do for one of these pieces, I spoke with a food chemist about some of the ways the various ingredients react with each other. As a good interview will sometimes do, our talk ventured off into other topics, and the scientist casually mentioned that the United States' food laws—regulations determining what can and cannot be used in food—are not always very strictly enforced.

I had firsthand knowledge of this. The FDA has produced a series of regulations called Standards of Identity, which are part of the US federal code and therefore have the force of law. In them, the FDA describes in minute detail what various foodstuffs are and what they are permitted to be. Ice cream, for instance, must contain at least 10 percent milk fat; butter can only be made from milk, cream, and salt; the moisture content of Limburger cheese must not exceed 51 percent; and so on.

EMULSIFIER

Sometimes, like oil and water or you and your mother-in-law, substances just refuse to mix. When placed in the same container they separate into layers, and any advantage that would come from mixing them doesn't happen. Unless you add an emulsifier: a substance that will encourage the suspension of one substance in another. Some emulsifiers work by reducing the surface tension between the two liquids. Others work by creating a film over one liquid, which forms into small globules that repel each other, thus causing them to remain suspended in the other liquid. Yet another type of emulsifier works by increasing the viscosity of one liquid, which helps to "trap" molecules of the other liquid in it.

I told the chemist that I was amazed to read the Standard of Identity for eggnog. The FDA makes it absolutely clear that eggnog may not contain any type of food coloring that makes it look as if there are more egg yolks in the eggnog than there actually are. This essentially means that any sort of yellow, or orange-and-yellow, food coloring should be banned from eggnog. This includes substances like the standard Yellow #5 food coloring, as well as more natural food colorings, such as the plant-based extracts annatto or turmeric. According to the FDA's Standard of Identity, those food colorings are disallowed in eggnog.

Yet, when I'd look at all the varieties of eggnog, I couldn't find a single brand that did *not* use some form of orange/yellow food coloring, in clear violation of the FDA's rule. I casually asked the food chemist how the dairy companies could get away with that.

The chemist got very, very quiet and immediately requested that our conversation be continued off the record. This is a journalistic agreement that means that nothing of what the journalist is told may be used in the story. The information is meant only for the education of the reporter. Going off the record usually indicates that the reporter is about to be handed (1) a load of crap or (2) a giant story. It can be hard to tell the difference.

When I agreed to go off the record, the scientist said, "This kind of thing happens all the time." I asked what she meant by that. She said that over the past fifteen years or so, the FDA has had its funding cut dramatically. Because of this, they pretty much have lost the ability to do standard proactive enforcement of many of their regulations. They spend too much of their time running around "putting out fires": dealing with an *E. coli* outbreak in hamburger, say, or tainted pharmaceuticals from China. And because of that, it has sort of become open season for those manufacturers who would like to bend the rules a little bit. She warned that she couldn't be certain that that was what was happening with eggnog, but she wouldn't be surprised if the dairy companies that make eggnog decided to push the rules a bit to see what they could get away with.

It sounds like a cliché, but the back of my scalp was literally tingling when she told me this. It was a flush of excitement, an intuition that I really, seriously might be onto a pretty big story. Was the entire dairy industry violating the law?

I couldn't use what the scientist told me, but I could use it as a springboard to do more of my own research. So I took it upon myself to call a university law professor who specialized in food law. I laid out the problem for him: according to government regulation 21CFR131.170, eggnog could not contain egglike food coloring, yet every eggnog I examined contained yellow or orange food coloring. I asked him what loopholes the dairy companies were using to clearly go against the letter and the spirit of this regulation. What's going on here?

I waited on the phone as I heard that clickety-clack of his computer keyboard as he looked up the regulations. He was quiet for what seemed like a long time (though probably was only about one minute), and then he said, "And you say that nearly every eggnog you've looked at contains a yellow or orange food coloring?" And I said yes, either Yellow #5 or annatto or turmeric.

The professor took a deep breath and let it out in a long

sigh. "If any of these companies hired me to be their adviser on food law, I would tell them to stop doing this immediately. Immediately."

"Why?"

"Because there is no loophole I can see. They're breaking the law."

I'd like to thank the Pulitzer committee for awarding me this prize in investigative reporting. Could this story really be serious? This professor was regularly hired by food companies to be an expert witness when the companies were brought to trial because of some violation they may have committed in the food laws. He told me that he generally worked on the side of the food companies against the government. Yet here he was, in essence, telling the food companies that they were wrong. What they were doing could not be defended in court. Their champion was telling them to give it up.

The story was getting bigger than I ever thought. If this expert witness was willing to come down against the food companies, then it was more than likely that they really were breaking the law. I had to take my inquiries even farther.

So I called a law firm that described themselves as top litigators against the FDA on behalf of food companies. These were the actual lawyers who went up against the government. They frequently won, and their attitude as winners showed.

When I identified myself as a reporter, the receptionist immediately passed me to one of the founders of the firm (and now partner emeritus). I kind of got the impression that he was more or less semiretired, and the firm trotted him out whenever someone from the media needed a quote about something. I identified myself to the man and once again laid out the entire story for him: 21CFR131.170 says no eggy food coloring, yet nearly every eggnog contains a yellow-orange food coloring. What was the deal?

The old man laid the phone on his desk—laid it on his desk without hitting the hold button. He had the voice of a very old man, but he displayed the mental energy, and the zeal for the fight, of a man half his age. He ordered his assistants to pull the relevant volumes off the shelves, because he wanted to look up 21CFR131.170 for himself. I then heard him ask for other tomes, all recited from memory. He barked orders and told people what to look up using obscure legal terminology. As the minutes dragged on, I could hear some of his younger minions report back to him, and I sat there at my desk with my headphone pressed up against my ear, straining mightily to overhear what they were saying. He asked more questions and barked more orders. I got the impression he was enjoying himself. I heard him pick up the phone off the desk.

"Young fella, you there?"

I said I was.

"You said you're a reporter?"

I said I was a writer for *Wired* magazine. He asked what the circulation was and I told him about three-quarters of a million people. I added that the magazine was part of the Condé Nast media empire. I had a subtle need to convey to him that I, too, was in the big leagues.

"Well, I'll tell you, if you write this up, and get it out there, it's going to have a big impact. A big impact."

When he said those words my skin tingled again, but in a different way. Before I was filled with the excitement of finding a big story. Now I was filled with the responsibility of finding a big story.

"What kind of big impact do you think it might have?" I asked.

"You said that the story's coming out around Thanksgiving?" the partner emeritus asked. "Well, if Condé Nast gives a big play, and if it gets picked up by other media, you could conceivably be responsible for getting the FDA to remove all eggnog from store shelves just before Christmas."

Ho-leee shiiiiiiiiiit. It was one thing to come up with a big story, to be talked about on *Fox and Friends* and interviewed by Rachel Maddow. It was an entirely different thing to be *the Grinch who destroyed Christmas.*

I needed some guidance, and fast. I called my editor at *Wired.*

Once again I laid out the entire story. I told him what the food chemist had hinted at, what the food professor had said, and what the food lawyer had said. I told him that we were potentially facing a story that might make a real but small change in the world, in a way that might get us all killed by angry mobs.

He questioned me relentlessly. Were the chemicals used to create the yellow color harmful in any way? I told him annatto and turmeric were totally natural vegetable-based colors. Yellow #5 had its detractors, some people who thought it wasn't safe, but it was still legal to use. Was I sure that annatto and turmeric were used to color egg yolks? I sent him links to various companies that encouraged chicken farmers to feed annatto and turmeric to their brood hens specifically to deepen the yellow color of their egg yolks. He asked if I had checked with the FDA. I told him I had spoken to their spokesperson several times, and now the poor guy was not returning my calls or e-mails anymore. He asked if I had checked with the various eggnog manufacturers. I told him that the Southern Comfort eggnog people were no longer returning my calls, and then I'd asked several other eggnog manufacturers, but they hadn't yet gotten back to me. He suggested that I check with the American Dairy Association and told me to keep him informed. He thought this was a good story.

I felt like Woodward and Bernstein and Scrooge all rolled into one. In America in the early years of the twenty-first century, I could seriously expect death threats if I did something to ruin Christmas. I was looking up the contact information for the American Dairy Association when I got a call from one of the eggnog manufacturers I had reached out to earlier.

"Mr. Di Justo, it's Charlie X from XXX Dairies, how are you today? I'm calling about that question you asked us yesterday, and boy, let me tell you, you gave us quite a scare. For a while there I really thought that we had been breaking the law."

What? He's happy? He says they're not breaking the law? But we know what the law says! Multiple people told me they were breaking the law! If they're not breaking the law, my big Pulitzer Prize–winning story is dead! "You're *not* breaking the law when you add yellow food coloring to eggnog?"

"No, we are not, thank goodness," Charlie said. "It's kind of complicated, so I suggest you call Athena at the American Dairy Association, and she can explain the whole thing to you. Here's her number."

I could barely speak. My story was dissolving in front of me. "I'll certainly do that," I said with a certainty I did not feel.

Athena at the American Dairy Association was efficiency personified. She asked me for my e-mail address, and she sent me a page from a 1981 *Federal Register,* the official journal of the United States government. In it, the government explained its ruling on the use of color additives in eggnog. The report explained that some eggnog manufacturers objected to the new rule, saying that the public has come to expect deep-yellow eggnog, a color that cannot be reached by pure egg yolk alone. Another manufacturer argued that different eggs (especially from chickens fed on annatto) have yolks that are different shades of yellow, and if egg farmers can tint their products to obtain a uniform appearance, eggnog manufacturers should be able to do the same.

The *Federal Register* document showed that ultimately, the FDA agreed with those arguments. The final sentence of that section of the document is as follows:

> Therefore, FDA is staying the effective date of that portion of § 131.170(e)(4) that prohibits the use of color additives that simulate the color of egg yolk, butterfat, or milkfat, pending the outcome of a public hearing.

In other words, the law against yellow was to remain on the books, but it would not be enforced until everyone got a chance to talk about it at a hearing.

I said to Athena, "Was the public hearing ever held?" Athena said she did not know.

"But that was more than thirty years ago!" I said. Athena agreed that it was, in fact, more than thirty years ago.

"All the people who were working at the FDA at that time, all the people who ever knew about this ruling, may be dead or retired by now," I said. Athena admitted that, yes, they might be dead or retired. "So the possibility of this hearing ever happening is essentially zero!" I cried. Athena maintained the tactful silence of the victorious for a long time, then asked if there was anything else she could do for me. I said no, there wasn't, and thanked her.

My story was dead, and for the worst reason. A law was put into place for a good cause, and it was being subverted in a way that made that subversion legal, in the most cynical way possible. The law was put on hold until further hearings could be held, and then those hearings were never held.

I was defeated. Later that night, I told my girlfriend everything that had happened that day: the excitement of getting a good story, the responsibility of realizing that my story might have serious real-world consequences, and the ultimate letdown of realizing that cynical flouting of the law extends all the way down to holiday foods.

She looked thoughtful for a moment, then said, "You've had a great lesson. You were nearly seduced by the Dark Side of Eggnog."

Spam with Bacon

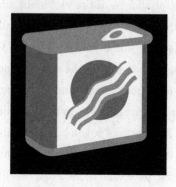

Pig, pig, pig, pig. And potato starch.

Pork with Ham

That's what the label says: "pork with ham." But aren't ham and pork the same thing? Is there a difference? According to the USDA, ham is the hind leg of a pig that's been preserved, colored, and flavored through a process known as curing, while pork is just "meat from hogs." According to Hormel, the pork in Spam is usually—but not always—chopped shoulder meat. What's certain is that the pig flesh is vacuum-sealed in the can while still raw and then cooked for three hours. Hormel says this gives Spam an indefinite shelf life, making it the go-to food for Depression-era Steinbeckian Okies, protein-hungry wartime Brits, and would-be subterranean nuclear holocaust survivors. (The company concedes that the flavor may change after three or more years on the shelf.)

Modified Potato Starch

Three hours of cooking in the can would tend to squeeze some of the moisture out of Spam. Modified potato starch to the rescue! The starch traps water molecules, binding that juicy goodness in the loaf. But modified how? It depends on how you want to use it: you can add sodium hypochlorite (a.k.a. liquid bleach, a.k.a. Clorox) to make the starch whiter, you can add octenyl succinic anhydride (a.k.a. a strange chemical) to increase its gel temperature, or you can add phosphoryl chloride to prevent the starch granules from swelling, to name just a few. However it is modified, Hormel credits this stuff—about 2 percent of each Spam mouthful—with maintaining "the delightful texture characteristic to SPAM©."

Sodium Nitrite

It's nothing but a sodium atom, a nitrogen atom, and two oxygen atoms. But meat processors love $NaNO_2$, because it inhibits the bug that causes botulism, adds flavor, and turns cured meat a "healthy" pink hue. The color magic happens when nitrites convert to nitric oxide (NO), which binds to the iron in muscle myoglobin to form a stable pigment when heated.

Salt

Cured meat? We didn't even know it was sick! Before the days of refrigeration, meats were preserved with salt, which denied water to bad microorganisms through the process of osmosis. Today, sodium nitrite serves that purpose, and plain old sodium chloride is mainly there for flavor. Spam with Bacon has far less sodium (1 percent by weight) than old-fashioned preserved meats (5 to 7 percent). Still, a 12-ounce can has about 3 grams, equivalent to 234 Ruffles potato chips. Salt isn't regulated by any government agency, because meat processors consider it to be self-limiting: Hormel isn't going to oversalt their products to the point of making them inedible.

Dextrose

USDA scientists discovered ninety years ago that some bacon cured with corn syrup turned dark black when cooked, and bacon cured with granulated sugar turned golden yellow (ewww), but bacon cured with dextrose came out just right, a crispy light brown. This is the result of the Maillard reaction, in which carbonyl groups from sugars combine with amines from meat and create melanoidins—brown nitrogenous pigments—that make food yummy and can kill the ulcer bacterium.

Sugar

Not absolutely necessary for curing meats, but oh, so good. The main use is for "flavor"—i.e., to counteract all that salt. Plus, it's the third point of the unholy trinity: the combination of fat, salt, and sugar that works on our brain's dopamine and opioid circuitry—the same sites that narcotics stimulate, setting up a reward feedback system in the brain that keeps us eating cured ham and bacon and Spam, and Spam, Spam, Spam, Spam, lovely Spam, wonderful Spaaaaaaammmm . . .

Bacon

"The cured belly of a swine carcass," says the USDA. "Mmmm, bacon," says most of America. Large-scale curing is usually done by injecting a brine solution into the belly of a butchered swine. The brine contains sodium erythorbate, an antioxidant that's chemically similar to vitamin C. But it's not here to prevent scurvy; instead it boosts the conversion of the sodium nitrite in bacon into nitric oxide, which minimizes the production of carcinogens when the pork belly is fried up. The brining increases the meat's weight by 12 percent, but a trip through a 128-degree smokehouse dries the bellies back to their original weight, ready to be combined with the pork and ham in this canned pig fest.

HOW USELESS E-MAIL BECAME SPAM

For many British children after World War II, Spam was meat. In an era in which candy, tea, cheese, and butter were still being rationed, Spam was plentiful and inexpensive, and it became almost a byword for the British themselves.

So it should come as no surprise that years later, some of those same British children, now grown-up with a television show of their own, would write a comedy sketch in which it is impossible to escape from Spam. Monty Python's Spam sketch lasts two minutes and six seconds, and mentions the word "Spam" 132 times, for a "Spam" density of nearly 63 "Spam"s per minute, or 1.05 "Spam"s per second.

So in the mid-1990s, when nonhackers discovered the Internet and realized they could flood our e-mail inboxes with poorly written advertisements, it was inevitable that computer professionals would use a Monty Python reference to describe stuff from which you could not escape. In fact, the word "spam" now so solidly means "unwanted e-mail" that during the research for this chapter, I searched for the various phrases built around the word "SPAM" so many times that Google thought I was a heavy-duty e-mail spammer and locked me out for about an hour.

All this attention had to have been a mixed blessing for Hormel. While we don't know the company's official response to the use of "spam" to mean "bad e-mail" (their PR person says, "SPAM® brand doesn't typically field questions related to this particular topic"), it's difficult to imagine that they were happy with it. Imagine the setting Hormel has to have on their own company's e-mail spam filters: how do you block bad stuff that has the same name as your top product?

This Is What You Put in Your Glass

Tap Water

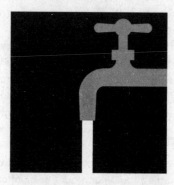

Radioactive particles, heavy metal poisoning, and rocket fuel juice all make for spigotty goodness!

Dihydrogen Monoxide

The International Union of Pure and Applied Chemistry calls it oxidane. You probably know it as H_2O. Essential for all life, it's the universal solvent as well as a biological lubricant and coolant. But when it comes out of your tap, this simple combination of hydrogen and oxygen atoms is often mixed with stuff that you might be less happy to swallow.

Fluoride

A massive international postwar Communist conspiracy to sap and impurify all of our precious bodily fluids. Alternately, it's part of a public health program to add either sodium fluoride, fluorosilicic acid, or sodium fluorosilicate to a region's drinking water supply. In your mouth, the fluoride mixes with hydroxyapatite, which is shed from teeth that are in the early stages of decay. The new compound, fluorapatite, gets redeposited onto the teeth, forming a harder coating that is more resistant to tooth decay. There are studies under way to fluoridate salt, flour, fruit juices, soup, sugar, milk . . . ice cream. *Ice cream, Mandrake, children's ice cream!*

Sulfate
This is a naturally occurring chemical that leaches into groundwater. It's not even necessarily a bad thing: some people (*cough* the French *cough*) drink high-sulfate mineral water at spas for its "cleansing" (i.e., laxative) effects. In public water supplies, the EPA recommends keeping it to 250 parts per million to minimize the sulfurous smell and taste. And, most likely, the cleansing effects.

Radionuclides
Millions of years ago, volcanic ash rich in uranium-238 blanketed what is now the gulf coast of Texas. Since then, the U-238 has made its way into aquifers, where it decays into radioactive isotopes like radium, thorium, and radon. In Houston, radiation levels in water have been measured as high as 16.9 picocuries per liter, well above the EPA maximum of 10 picocuries. (Yes, that unit of measure for radioactivity is named after Marie Curie—a fine tribute to a glowing career.) At least Houston's municipal water supply is specially treated to mitigate the excess radiation; thousands of people drinking untreated well water in the region can regularly ingest much higher levels of alpha particles, the stuff that actually causes radiation poisoning in the body.

Trihalomethanes
Like fluorine and bromine, chlorine belongs to the group of intensely reactive halogen elements—so reactive due to their electronegativity that they're the home wreckers of the periodic table, capable of breaking up many molecules (like ozone in the stratosphere). That makes chlorine great for killing microorganisms in water, which is a good thing. But chlorine

(and the other halogens) can also combine with organic matter to form molecules called trihalomethanes—three halogen atoms attached to what used to be a methane molecule. These monstrosities damage your DNA and liver, and may cause cancer.

N-nitrosodimethylamine

There's no maybe about this stuff—research labs have actually used this to *induce* cancer in rats with as little as one injection. But relax: NDMA can be formed accidentally, as a by-product of water purification with chlorine or chloramine. You might also accidentally ingest it if you live near a Cold War–era military base; it was found in ICBM fuel that leached into the ground. Riverside County, California, home of much of the nation's rocket and missile development, has measured levels of this stuff as high as twelve parts per trillion—four times the state's target limit.

Lead

New York City boasts about the quality of its drinking water, but that upstate freshness means nothing if the water travels through some of the oldest pipes in the country. (Even new "lead-free" pipes can be 8 percent lead.) New York's legendary soft water readily absorbs Pb, which can cause developmental disabilities and neurological problems. City authorities are required to take steps when levels hit fifteen parts per billion, and they commonly see rates as high as nineteen parts per billion; as recently as July 2012, a water monitoring station in Tribeca hit a peak of twenty-six parts of lead per billion.

Chloramines

You know how ammonia labels say, DO NOT MIX WITH BLEACH— and bleach labels say, DO NOT MIX WITH AMMONIA? Municipal water utilities, in their zeal to kill microorganisms, have been ignoring that advice for the past hundred years. Sure, the result is cleaner water, plus a few parts per million of this stuff—a compound that can damage red blood cells in mice and some humans.

Bromate

No, it's not some chill dude that you share your Old Spice with. This potential carcinogen is another water-purification practice gone awry. When water containing bromine ions from natural mineral deposits is purified with ozone (O_3), bromate (BrO_3) is born. And bromate poisoning is not some theoretical possibility: in 2008 the LA water authority had to drain two reservoirs that were bromate contaminated.

[BACKSTORY]

Another great one, inspired by the simplest action: taking a drink of water.

My girlfriend is a health nut, except when it comes to chocolate. New York City has some of the best and cleanest water in the country, yet she still insists on using a water-filter pitcher to keep cold water in the fridge. One night, as I was sleepily manipulating the water pitcher and filter trying to get a drink of water in the middle of the night, I started thinking: *Exactly what does she expect to filter out of the water?*

That led me to a wild search that stopped for a time at the Environmental Working Group. They're an NGO that produces really good, interesting data about the environment. A few years back they had produced a report about the "dirtiest" drinking water in the US. Most of the data had come from 2004 or 2005, which meant that it was time for us to update their findings.

The EPA was supposed to have completed a system by which you could visit their website and pull up the latest water quality report for any municipal water system that re-

---

LIQUID
A liquid consists of a group of molecules held together by weak intermolecular bonds, like the last remaining workers in a dying company. This differs from a gas, in which the molecules are not held together at all, or a solid, in which the bonds holding the molecules together are strong enough to keep them rigid. The liquid's weak bonds allow it to flow—that is, to deform when stress is applied—and it also lets the liquid take the shape of the container it is in.

ports to the EPA. Unfortunately, due to other circumstances (budget cuts? Political inertia? Direct obstruction? We may never know), that database system didn't exist. No matter; since these reports were produced by each local water system, I went around to the websites of various cities and towns looking for their EPA water quality reports.

If you've got an afternoon, I highly recommend you try this. Go to a city's website, search around until you find "water department" or something like that, and then look for something called an annual report. The quality of each of these reports varies immensely. New York City's annual water quality report is a glossy multipage pamphlet that looks like a prospectus to invest in water. For some other cities, the report is a single PDF document that has been output from a spreadsheet.

Once I had collected about twenty of these reports from all over the country, I started looking for commonalities. When I found more than one municipality with the same problem with a particular water contaminant, onto the list went that contaminant.

This Is What You Put in Your Mouth

Vita Coco Coconut Water

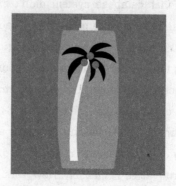

Endosperm. No, really. Endosperm.

Water

Coconut water is, in fact, mostly water: at least 94-95 percent pure H_2O. (This is not to be confused with coconut milk, which is made by blending minced white coconut flesh with coconut water.) Since a coconut is a giant seed, the remaining substances in coconut water are what make this the intracellular fluid of plant reproduction. Yes, that's right: when you drink coconut water you're drinking liquid coconut endosperm.

N[6]-furfuryladenine

Also known as kinetin, this is one of the cytokinins, a family of plant hormones (yes, plants have hormones too) that induce plant cell division. This is exactly the kind of chemical you'd expect to find inside a giant plant seed: something to make the seed grow into a tree when conditions are right. So how come it also has strong antiaging effects on human skin cells? Scientists are still working on that. But they do know that kinetin doesn't necessarily increase the *life span* of skin cells—it just holds off the onset of cellular and biochemical characteristics associated with cellular aging. It's sort of like botox, with an expiration date.

Gibberellins

It may sound like a cartoon name, but these things are real. They're a group of plant hormones generally found in the fastest-growing parts of the plant—root tips, young fruits, and germinating seeds. Their wonder-working power is astounding: dwarf plants can be made tall, and summer plants can be made to flower in winter conditions by the injection of one or another of the gibberellins. Unfortunately, if you're drinking coconut water in the hopes of rejuvenating yourself, these plant juices don't seem to have any effect, good or bad, on humans. The only *possible* benefit to the human body that we've heard of comes from 13-chlorine-3, 15-dioxy-gibberellic acid methyl ester (GA-13315), a gibberellin derivative with known antitumor properties. As always, further studies are needed to determine if this could really be an effective anticancer drug.

Abscisic Acid

YAPH (Yet Another Plant Hormone). If gibberellins promote growth in the springtime, abscisic acid (ABA) is the hormone of winter. It inhibits growth and suppresses cell division, which is exactly what you want in a plant that's about to sleep through the snowy months. (In fact, the technical term for leaves falling off trees in autumn is "abscission," and ABA is partly to blame.) It's also a stress hormone. If the plant experiences a drought, ABA will cause the pores in the plant's leaves—the stomata—to close up, preventing moisture loss. Unlike gibberellins, however, abscisic acid does have a pretty interesting effect on mammals like us: it is an effective anti-inflammatory and can ameliorate symptoms of type II diabetes. But don't think you can go off your diabetes meds in favor of nut juice.

AMINO ACID

Take an amine group ($-NH_2$) and an acid group (in this case carboxylic acid, $-COOH$), and attach them to another molecule. You've just made an amino acid, the functional unit of proteins (and commonly known as "the building blocks of life"). There are about five hundred amino acids known to scientists today, but only twenty of them (known as "standard" amino acids) can be encoded by our DNA to make proteins. In addition to their role as protein builders, amino acids are used to make neurotransmitters, hemoglobin, and genetic material. In the factory, they can be made into artificial sweeteners—aspartame is built around the amino acid phenylalanine—and biodegradable plastics.

· ·

PART TWO

THIS IS WHAT YOU
DON'T PUT IN YOUR MOUTH

Axe Deodorant

I'm too sexy for my flammable aluminized crosspolymer fluid.

Aluminum Zirconium Tetrachlorohydrex Gly

Nearly every antiperspirant has a mineral—usually aluminum—that dissolves into the skin with the first beads of sweat. This active ingredient causes underarm pores to swell shut, which stops more sweat from seeping out. And it kills odor-causing bacteria. Of course, a high dose of aluminum (far more than you're likely to get from a swipe of antiperspirant) can aggravate renal disease. So Unilever is taking no chances: the label suggests that kidney patients consult a doctor before enjoying the Axe effect. Not convinced rubbing metal under your arms is the way to go? You could always try the hippest new antiperspirant trend: Botox. Injected into the pits, the toxins keep you totally dry (if a little tingly).

Cyclopentasiloxane

This is a flammable silicone crosspolymer fluid (the silicon and oxygen atoms alternate to form a ring) with attached hydrogen atoms and methyl groups. The silicone evaporates quickly and helps spread the active ingredient. Don't worry; as flammable as it is, it probably won't catch fire under your arms.

PPG-14 Butyl Ether

"PPG" stands for "polypropylene glycol," one of those wondrous substances that can be made into anything—from wound dressings to lipstick. A mild skin irritant, PPG-14BE is an antistatic agent. So why is it here? Perhaps because dry armpits sometimes build up static cling. Then again, it's also sometimes used as an insecticide, in case you're attracting flies.

Stearyl Alcohol

A waxy solid, this crumbly stuff works in most cosmetics as a dry lubricant and moisturizer. Here it keeps the product from foaming up when rubbed vigorously across the skin. (After all, who needs a case of pit suds when you're trying to impress the ladies?) Oh, and it makes your underarm hair soft and shiny.

Hydrogenated Castor Oil

More crumbly stuff. This oil is used in many industries as a water-resistant wax and sometimes in hot-melt glue. Think of it here as Armor All for the underarm—it keeps moisture from collecting under your arms.

Fragrance

The secret to the Axe effect is, well, a secret. Unilever claims the scent will drive the ladies crazy. It smells like a junior high school dance to us.

Talc

Baby powder is safe, right? At least for grown men. Turns out, some studies suggest there's a link between genital talc use and ovarian cancer. So keep your pits out of your lady's pants.

BHT

This antioxidant keeps the butyls and stearyls and castor oil from reacting with oxygen and losing their effectiveness.

Colored-Flame Artificial Logs

*A hunk-a, hunk-a burning . . . wax. And sawdust.
And snowmelter. And birdseed, even . . .*

Paraffin

About half of the weight of a fire log is wax, usually inexpensive petroleum-based paraffin. It serves as a fuel, a binder for the other ingredients, and a structure for the log itself. Essentially, you're burning a giant sideways candle in your fireplace.

Wood Particles

Even though the whole point of a fake log is not to be a real log, fake logs are still about 40 percent real plant cellulose. (Duraflame, just to use one example, started as a way for California Cedar Products to make use of leftover sawdust.) Typical cellulosic material might be bark, cardboard, peanut shells, or coffee grounds. Even the log's paper wrapper doubles as tinder to get the fire going.

Nonpetroleum Waxes

Some newer fire logs claim to be biosustainable. They still use wax, but instead of stuff that's pumped out of the ground, they get their wax by stripping the leaves off rain forest plants (to get carnauba wax), chopping down pine trees (to get "tall oil," a liquid rosin), or slaughtering defenseless animals (to get tallow).

Lithium Carbonate

Flame is exciting to both people and atoms. On the quantum scale, fired-up electrons absorb energy, jump to a higher orbit, and then come crashing down, emitting photons of light at specific wavelengths. Burning Li_2CO_3 creates flames at a wavelength of 652 nanometers, which we perceive as an exotic red.

Potassium Chloride

Salt substitute, sidewalk-ice melter, and the "lethal" part of a lethal injection, KCl burns with a delicate blue-violet flame.

Copper Chloride/Copper Carbonate

Hard-core hackers who etch their own circuit boards at home swear by copper chloride; nothing eats unmasked copper like $CuCl_2$. Copper carbonate, $CuCO_3$, is the green coating on old pennies and the Statue of Liberty. The copper electrons in both chemicals emit electric-blue light in a fire.

Barium Carbonate

This rat poison, when set alight, produces the pale apple-green flames (with a wavelength of 589 nanometers) that seem to be the color most people associate with color logs.

Birdseed

Natural logs (especially pine) crackle as the moisture and oils in the wood reach their boiling points and "pop." To duplicate this effect, some fire logs contain between 2 and 6 percent birdseed (hemp, millet, coriander, or flax), which is also prone to pop when burned.

Metallurgical Coke

Coke, in this context, is coal with its volatile components—water, gases, coal tar—baked away. It can be ground into four-millimeter particles that sputter when heated.

Hollow Spheres

When these glass, ceramic, or polymer orbs are heated, enormous pressure builds up from the little bit of moisture or air inside. Eventually the outer shells explode—just like the rest of us during the holidays when trapped with our families—mimicking the snapping, crackling, and popping of a real log.

My favorite little tidbit is the birdseed. It is so simple it is positively brilliant! They act like little popcorn kernels embedded in fake wood, popping at pseudorandom times!

But my favorite unknown part of this story is my discovery of W. Hughes Brockbank, renaissance man of the American West. He was a miner, a real estate developer, and an education pioneer, and spent two terms in the Utah state legislature and four terms as a state senator. He also ran a profitable janitorial supply company, and once he sued the governor of Utah to preserve a legislator's right to sell janitorial supplies to the state legislature without having to worry about messy things like conflict-of-interest laws. He was a member of the Utah board of regents, and he served on educational commissions in the Nixon and Reagan administrations.

But for all those accomplishments, W. Hughes Brockbank will be forever remembered in these pages as the man who, all the way back in 1969, first patented the process of making an artificial fireplace log that produced colored flames.

REDUCTION

This is pretty much the opposite of oxidation. Just as oxidation is thought of as adding an oxygen atom to a molecule, reduction can be thought of as losing an oxygen atom or adding a hydrogen atom. As the definition of "oxidation" became more refined to mean losing electrons, "reduction" came to mean the act of accepting electrons. If you remember what we said about acids, since they accept electrons in their reactions, they get reduced, compared to bases, which get oxidized.

Bausch & Lomb Renu Contact Lens Cleaner Solution

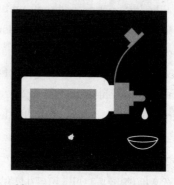

Crocodile tears? No, just fake human ones.

Dymed

Contact lens cleaning solution has to disinfect an object that comes into contact with the eyeball without burning your eyes when you pop the lenses in. Dymed (polyaminopropyl biguanide), derived from the French lilac, is an antimicrobial agent that attaches to bad little bugs and rips open their cell membranes, letting their guts spill out. Fortunately for your eyeballs, it only works on single-celled organisms, and it rinses away cleanly without binding to the lens, so it doesn't come into contact with your eye.

Hydranate

Known by chemists as hydroxyalkylphosphonate, it removes protein deposits, eliminating the hassle of a separate enzyme treatment. The eye's lubricating fluid contains mucus protein, which over time can build up and cloud your vision like a snot cataract. Hydranate is an ophthalmically safe detergent that traps the mucus molecules and lifts them off the surface of the lens.

Boric Acid

It's a fire retardant, a nuclear-reaction controller, cockroach powder, and the stuff that turns silicone oil into Silly Putty. Grandma knew it as an antiseptic eyewash; here it's also a pH buffer. But boric acid has been tagged by the Feds as an infant-killing poison. There's only a dash in Renu, so don't worry—unless you experience one of the more memorable symptoms of boric acid toxicity: blue-green vomit.

Edetate Disodium

This commonly used compound sequesters metallic ions (calcium from tears or possibly particles from air pollution) that might otherwise react with the lens.

Sodium Chloride

Since soft lenses are liquid permeable, you want to make sure that your cleaning fluids are as osmotically close to tears as possible. That calls for a pinch of salt—otherwise, the lenses would dry out. Add too much, of course, and your lenses will suck all the moisture out of your eyes, get oversaturated, and start to weep. Creepy.

Poloxamine

A very gentle detergent that ensnares lipids so they can be washed away. It is a block copolymer made of multiple oxyethylene and oxypropylene segments, which is just a bunch of scientific words you don't need to worry about. The really cool thing is that the structure of poloxamines makes them work almost like keys that unlock very specific cell membranes. For this reason, they're also used in gene therapy as an alternative to artificial viruses for carrying DNA into cells, and for carrying anticancer drugs directly into tumors and not the surrounding cells. That doesn't have anything to do with contact lenses, but it's cool to know.

Sodium Borate

More widely recognized under the alias borax, it's the same crystalline alkali dust found in Death Valley. It's added to Renu as a buffering agent, keeping the solution at a comfy pH of 6.5 to 7.8. Since your tears are a perfectly neutral pH 7.0, you'll never have to utter the words "Ahhh, my eyes!"

CoverGirl LashBlast Luxe Mascara

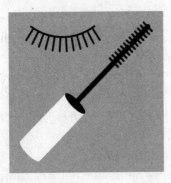

Iron(III) oxide to give you those "magnetic" eyes.

Disteardimonium Hectorite

This molecule is shaped like a squid with a nitrogen body and fatty-alcohol tentacles. Hectorite, a powdery volcanic clay, coats the tentacles, giving them bulk and a positive charge. Since hair has a negative static electrical charge, the molecule sticks to lashes, making them seem thicker.

Propylene Carbonate

A "safe" and environmentally friendly solvent, this keeps the other ingredients from separating. It's a polar molecule, meaning that each end of it has a different electrical charge that attracts and repels different materials. But it is also aprotic, meaning it can't release protons, which could react with those other components in the mascara.

Iron(III) Oxide

Don't wear mascara to a cranial MRI! There is so much of this dark black metallic pigment here (as much as 10 percent by weight) that its ferromagnetic properties can screw up diagnostic images, creating a splotch over your eye that the doctor will interpret as melanoma. Why is it here? Because "shiny."

Panthenol

Dry, brittle lashes can break off, taking up to nine months to grow back. The jury is out as to whether panthenol makes hair grow, but everyone agrees that lashes can at least be conditioned and moisturized by this precursor to vitamin B5, making them less susceptible to snapping in two.

Paraffin and Carnauba Wax

Paraffin comes from a petroleum refinery, carnauba comes from the Brazilian rain forest, but both these waxes help carry the various pigments as well as artificially lengthen and thicken the eyelashes.

Triethanolamine

This stuff is a thickener and emulsifier and also lowers the surface tension of the mascara, allowing it to adhere to the brush and the lashes.

Ammonium Acrylates Copolymer

Listed as "practically nonirritating" when tested on the eyeballs of live rabbits, this emulsifier and pigment disperser gives a nice glossy coating to the eyelash and enhances flexibility under the weight of all that iron oxide.

Bismuth Oxychloride

Another pigment with strange magnetic properties. Thanks to variations in the thickness of the oxide layer, this compound creates that shimmery pearlescent look on each eyelash. (This effect used to come from guanine, which is probably how the "bat poop in mascara" rumor got started.)

Dichromium Trioxide

A dark green pigment with odd paramagnetic effects like its cousin CrO_2, a coating for audiotape. Highly resistant to heat, light, and chemicals, this stuff could theoretically be formulated to make your eyelashes reflect infrared light—just like the best military camouflage.

. . . .

SURFACE TENSION

The intermolecular forces that hold a liquid together are usually distributed all around the molecules and are therefore weak enough to allow the liquid to flow. But at the juncture between the surface of the liquid and the air above it, the molecules do not have intermolecular forces distributed all around them. The forces pull together on the liquid side but not on the air side, creating a very strong boundary. This tension is what keeps water droplets together and what allows you to very carefully fill a glass higher than its brim. Unfortunately, surface tension is a drawback when you deliberately want objects to get wet, such as in a washing machine. Detergents are specifically designed to counteract surface tension and let water penetrate into clothing, the better to get the dirt out. Surface tension also can occur between two different types of liquid that do not mix, such as oil and water.

[BACKSTORY]

W hat's Inside" can go a long time between researching products that are commonly thought of as "women's." So it was exciting to get into the workings of mascara, considering it had been at least twenty-five years since I last wore the stuff. (Saturday nights. New Rochelle Proctor's movie theater. Midnight performances of *The Rocky Horror Picture Show*. Me as Dr. Frank-N-Furter. No, no pictures exist.) How had it changed?

I started examining mascara ingredient lists, and mascara formulas, and mascara patents, and it occurred to me that with all these metallic compounds, mascara ought to be affected by a magnet. Could this be true? Had no one noticed this before?

I asked some friends if they felt any strange magnetic attraction when they wore mascara. Then I realized that the question was too vague. I asked them if they had ever stuck kitchen magnets to their eyelashes while wearing mascara. They told me to go away and stop bothering them.

I asked my girlfriend if she had any mascara. She doesn't need (and doesn't really use) makeup, so I wasn't sure if I had ever seen it on her. She thought she might have one tube, in the back of a drawer. While she dug it out, I found the rare-earth magnets I had salvaged from the last hard drive I destroyed. These are powerful magnets that can attract even the smallest amount of ferrous metal; if there was anything magnetic about mascara, these magnets would find out. We delicately brought the mascara and the magnets together. . . .

And the bottle of mascara stuck to the magnets!

Diamond Strike Anywhere Matches

A plastic explosive stuck on a splinter of cloned tree.

Aspen

This soft white wood is easy to cultivate: clusters of aspen trees are often gigantic single organisms, spreading over many acres. An aspen forest is, quite literally, a clone army of the same tree. Since the organism is so large, cutting down part of the forest usually results in new growth sprouting out of the soil after harvesting. Aspen doesn't burn well—the Forest Service recommends planting it as a firebreak due to its low flammability—making for a perfect slow-burning, non-fingertip-singeing matchstick.

Potassium Dichromate

This strong oxidizer in the match head is highly combustible. Diamond, the sole US manufacturer of strike-anywhere matches, won't say what it does, preferring to keep the role of $K_2Cr_2O_7$ a secret. Our bet: it accelerates burn rate.

Potassium Chlorate

It's a source of emergency air on planes, submarines, and spacecraft. In those places, this chemical is usually called an oxygen candle: it actually gives off breathable air when it is ignited. When it is mixed with wax, this stuff makes a great plastic explosive. When mixed with sulfur, phosphorus, and the kind of heat you get from, say, friction, it's very unstable and liable to burst into flame. Just like a matchstick.

Phosphorus Sesquisulfide

P_4S_3 also ignites easily by friction. It burns itself out instantly after the match is lit but generates enough heat to ignite the aspen shank. Diamond released its patent for P_4S_3 matches in 1911 so competitors could stop using an extremely dangerous alternative: explosive white phosphorous.

Monoammonium Phosphate

A compound found in some dry chemical fire extinguishers, MAP melts at 374 degrees Fahrenheit and smothers the fire. What is it doing in a fire stick? Match makers soak the wood with a solution of this stuff to make sure that when you blow the match out, it stays out: melted MAP smothers any afterglow.

Ground or Powdered Glass

First, it roughens the texture of the match head, helping to create friction wherever you strike it. Second, it melts under fire but cools and fuses quickly when you blow the flame out, keeping ash from falling.

FIRE

Think about it. With the invention of the match, for the first time in history humans had the ability to create fire whenever and wherever they wanted it, and—this is the killer app part—with a minimum of effort.

When I was a kid, I was fascinated with the movie *Quest for Fire*, about a tribe of movie Neanderthals who get raided by a neighboring tribe and have their only source of fire extinguished. Since their tribe lacks the knowledge of how to produce fire, the elders send three warriors (the Hero, the Lancer, and the Comic Relief) out to find some: they're on a Quest for Fire.

They soon run into the actress Rae Dawn Chong, who is a member of a more advanced Cro-Magnon tribe who have discovered simple technologies like gourds and advanced spears but have not yet invented clothes. After many adventures with cannibals and woolly mammoths and naked Rae, the warriors return to their tribe to show them a skill they learned from Chong's more advanced people—how to start fires with a hand drill.

A hand drill is sort of like rubbing two sticks together, but much more elegantly. It works by taking a pointed stick, called the spindle, and spinning its point between the palms against a flat surface, called the hearth, which is also surrounded by tinder, a collection of dried leaves, grass, or fungus that catches fire easily. The intense friction concentrated at the point of the stick is usually enough to produce an ember in the tinder, which can then be nursed into a full flame. It sounds like a simple task, but getting the right spindle, hearth, and tinder together is not easy, and—as seen in the last scene of the movie—it can take some practice to actually get a fire going.

By about 3300 BC, contemporaries of Ötzi the Iceman, a Neolithic herder whose preserved body was found on an Austrian mountain glacier, were making fire using a wood-handled flint knife and a lump of naturally occurring iron sulfide. Striking the flint, a hard variant of quartz, against the iron sulfide lump made tiny bits of iron sulfide, which can ignite spontaneously in the air and set the tinder alight. Like the hand-drill method, the process isn't easy: in *A Tale of Two Cities* Charles Dickens explains the process and adds that with a bit of luck, one could get a fire going in about five minutes.

Why were a Neolithic herdsman and a Victorian writer using the same method to start fires? Because in the five thousand years separating the two, popular fire making hadn't really advanced much. Yes, alchemical research with boiling urine in the 1600s led to the discovery of white phosphorus, which ignites on contact with the air, but this wasn't a viable solution for fire starting; first, it required huge vats of urine, which is something only a few hobbyists had, and second, you could probably just get your flame from the fire used to boil the urine, anyway.

But those researchers had let the phosphorous genie out of the specimen cup. Soon, alchemists realized that phosphorus could be mined from rocks, which lowered costs and solved their piddling supply-chain problem. By the early 1800s scientists had found a way to start a fire with a combination of potassium chlorate, sulfur, and sugar. In 1805 this became the first self-igniting match, invented in Paris. It was a nice bit of lab work but was impractical in the field; to work it you had to dip the match into a small bottle of sulfuric acid, which few people were willing to carry around with them in the hopes that someone would ask them for a light.

April Fresh Downy Fabric Softener

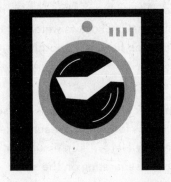

*Stop. Stop reading this right now. You do not want
to know. Stop. Just move along. Now . . .*

Dihydrogenated Tallow Dimethyl Ammonium Chloride

This substance is derived from rendered fat from cattle, sheep,
or horses. Just boil it down and mix with ammonium (NH_4). After
a series of chemical steps, out comes a quaternary ammonium
compound, or quat—a positive ion in which the hydrogen is
replaced by long-chain organic molecules. Quats effectively coat
your clothing with a thin layer of lipids, making the fibers soft
to the touch. These fats also make fabric a bit less absorbent,
so don't use on towels or cloth diapers. One good effect from
ionized horse fat: the positive charge neutralizes static electricity.

1-Methyl-1-tallowamidoethyl-2-tallowimidazolinium Methylsulfate

If you look in the middle of the chemical's name, you'll see
the letters "imidazolin." They are a family of biologically active
carbon-nitrogen rings that act as decongestants, antipsychotics,
or insecticides (which makes honeybees deranged and leads to
colony collapse). Here, however, it's nothing more exotic than
another quat.

Calcium Chloride

These water-absorbing crystals are in everything from road deicers to food additives. It's here because left on their own, the two quats (above) tend to spontaneously group into spherical fatty globules; CaCl draws water out of them by osmosis, keeping the goo flowing smoothly.

PEG 8000

This is polyethylene glycol. The "8000" is this substance's molecular weight; in this formulation, each molecule weighs as much as a small protein. Here, it's an emulsifier, keeping the fats and other liquids from separating on the shelf.

Kathon CG

Also known by the catchy moniker 5-chloro-2-methyl-3-isothiazolinone. When you pack so much animal fat into one place, you're essentially serving up a giant jug of microbial nutrient medium. Without powerful antimicrobials like isothiazolinones, April Fresh would quickly turn into August Rancid.

Perfume

The sizzle that sells the steak: research shows that scent—locked into the clothing fibers by the fatty coating—is the main reason consumers choose one detergent or fabric softener over another. This might be changing with the development of perfumeless and clear variants.

Ethanol and Isopropanol

Downy is shipped year-round and isn't always stored at room temperature. If the quat cocktail were to drop below freezing, it would thicken and need to be dissolved in water. (Think of the way an egg white goes from liquid to solid when it is heated and retains that solidity even after it cools. Similar thing happens here, only in reverse.) Alcohols act as antifreeze to keep this product from solidifying into a pitcher of lard.

. . . .

Deionized Water

This is added as a preservative for the various quats in the bottle. It also eliminates any ferric ions (dissolved iron) present in your laundry water, which can yellow some fabrics.

. . . .

[BACKSTORY]

Horse fat? *Horse fat?* On my clothes??

When you think of your basic needs, you may think shelter, food, and clothing are at the top of the list. It's quite possible that you can still really be happy if your clothes aren't "touchably soft."

In researching this piece, I discovered that fabric softener started out, like so many products, as a response to a problem no one had. Old-fashioned laundry soap, being made of fats, tended to leave behind a thin film of lipids on the washed clothes; newfangled laundry detergents didn't leave that film, resulting in clothes that were marginally less soft. At roughly the same time in history, chemists came up with quaternary ammonium compounds, which were essentially easily controllable lipids. So detergent companies replaced laundry soap with a product that didn't leave fatty scum on your clothes, then invented a product designed specifically to leave fatty scum on your clothes. This is what you call progress.

And to what end? Fabric softener, by coating your clothes with a thin layer of fat, cuts down the absorbancy of your towels, rags, and cloth diapers, precisely the reason you bought them in the first place!

Febreze

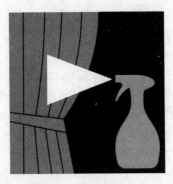

It's like smothering bad smells with little sugary hoops of love.

Nitrogen

When Freon and other chlorofluorocarbons were found in the 1970s to be dangerous to the ozone layer, aerosol manufacturers scrambled to find alternative propellants. Some changed their product to work with a pump spray, others moved to hydrocarbon propellants like butane, and others settled on everyday gases like CO_2 or nitrogen, which are part of our atmosphere. Why did it take so long for aerosol manufacturers to use an obviously harmless gas like N_2? Because nitrogen has always had less spraying power than other gases and is pretty much a last resort.

. . . .

Cyclodextrin

The odor eliminator, and the raison d'être for Febreze. Cyclodextrins, as their name implies, are glucose molecules ("dextrins") arranged in a closed loop like a doughnut ("cyclo"). There could be anywhere from six to twelve glucose units in the circles, arranged so that the inside of the doughnut is heavy with hydrogen molecules, making the interior fairly hydrophobic, or repulsive to water. This arrangement means that cyclodextrins act almost like soap: the interior of the loop absorbs stinky organic molecules, making them incapable of floating up your nose.

Purified Water

The patent for Febreze is adamant: water (they call it the "aqueous solution") is necessary to keep the smells and the cyclodextrins in solution: Febreze wouldn't do a good job of trapping bad smells without its water. Why must the water be purified? Because microorganisms such as *E. coli* are found in some water supplies, and because cyclodextrins are basically little sugary loops of bacteria food. Plus, did you know that plain water has odor-eating qualities? The authors of the Febreze patent believe that water "solubilizes and depresses the vapor pressure of polar low molecular weight organic molecules, thus reducing their odor intensity."

Alcohol

This is a drying agent. You don't want to sit around in a wet Febreze puddle, do you?

Various Perfume Blends

Procter & Gamble is quite clear on the concept: the delicate fragrance used in Febreze is *not* meant to be a perfume that covers up odors. As such, it's only in here from about 0.005 percent to about 0.2 percent by weight—hardly enough to stink up the joint. Instead, you should think of this soupçon of scent as a signal that Febreze is on the job, removing the malodor from fabrics. It's the olfactory equivalent of the five signal bars on your phone, only for your nose. For your pleasure, P & G scientists included on their website a page-and-a-half-long list (in tiny type) of ninety-nine different fragrance chemicals they suggest using, either solo or in combination. That makes for 9.332622×10^{155} different smells.

Dialkyl Sodium Sulfosuccinate

Scientists call this a solubilizing aid, a substance that helps disperse Febreze around your room. The best solubilizers are surfactants, or surface-active agents, also known as detergents. This is an anionic surfactant, which has a negative electrical charge. Since similar electrical charges repel each other, the negatively charged Febreze droplets will spread more effectively through the room.

Benzisothiazolinone

This stuff protects the product from microbial contamination. As we said, cyclodextrins are microscopic sugar loops, and many microorganisms would find them to be a nutritious breakfast. Add water, and the whole thing is a formula for germ soup. Since cyclodextrins probably can't be purified 100 percent against some bacteria (e.g., *Bacillus thuringiensis*) and fungi (e.g., *Aspergillus ustus*), the patent calls for generous use (in the range of about 0.1 percent) of a broad-spectrum microbial that goes after both fungi and bacteria, as long as it doesn't stain fabric. When the patent says that this product is "not for use on human skin," that's because the European Union found that about 10 percent of people report skin irritation when testing this stuff.

[BACKSTORY]

Febreze has long been the Holy Grail of those of us who look at ingredient lists. For years, it was next to impossible to find anything about what made Febreze tick. Part of this is due to the trend of inventors (or patent lawyers) being increasingly vague in the way they name their patents. In the 1950s, say, a patent for artificial snow would be called "Artificial Snow." These days, patents for artificial snow are called something like "Pigmented Spray Texture Material Compositions, Systems, and Methods." How could you expect to find that if you're looking for artificial snow?

This problem applies even more strongly to Febreze, because of the problems Procter & Gamble had defining the product. They initially announced Febreze in 1998, calling it a "Fabric Refresher," to eliminate unwanted household odors

ODOR MOLECULES

- amines, which can smell like ammonia or decaying fish
- acids, which can smell vinegary, acrid, or sweaty
- aldehydes, which can smell "green"—like grass, flowers, or spices
- ketones, which can smell from musky to breadlike
- phenolics, a sweet "medicinal" smell
- polycyclics, whose smells run the gamut from musky to burned
- indoles, which are the fecal family of smells
- thiols, which smell garlicky, asparagusy, and gassy
- mercaptans, which smell skunky

from soft surfaces. It was a flop—most people were used to their own household odors and didn't see a need to get rid of them. As Charles Duhigg reported in the *New York Times Magazine* ("How Companies Learn Your Secrets," February 16, 2012), P & G interviewed and reinterviewed consumers, videotaped their housecleaning routines, and hired researchers and a Harvard Business School professor to figure out what they were doing wrong. The breakthrough came when they realized that consumers were using the product as a pleasant treat at the end of the cleaning ritual, not as a fixer of bad smells. Procter & Gamble quickly revamped their advertising, and Febreze sales took off. As Duhigg puts it, "And so Febreze, a product originally conceived as a revolutionary way to destroy odors, became an air freshener used once things are already clean."

All very well for P & G, but what about our problems? What are the ingredients of Febreze? That was still a corporate secret. Until suddenly it wasn't. Sometime in 2009, P & G put up their www.pgproductsafety.com website, which listed all the ingredients for all their products.

This was a fascinating development. I (and many others) had been pestering them since 2006 to be more open about the ingredients in their products. Did the popularity of a monthly magazine column, along with countless other blogs, finally bring them to a tipping point where P & G management judged that it was better to let the information out than to keep it a mystery? Or did they realize that they could probably easily withstand whatever revelations I discovered?

No matter: our long, anxious wait was finally over. Now the world would know the secrets of Febreze!

This Is What You Put in Your Tires

Fix-A-Flat

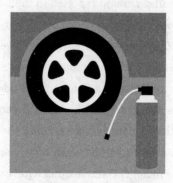

Rubber and air and testicle poison.

Tetrafluoroethane

A type of fluorocarbon that doesn't deplete the ozone layer,
TFE is found in everything from cryogenic tissue kits (when
research scientists cut organs and other bits out of laboratory
animals for study, they almost always give the excised tissue
a blast with a compressed jet of tetrafluoroethane to freeze
it instantly) to car air conditioners. In this product it's used as
a tire inflator, a drying agent, and a propellant for the other
ingredients. Unfortunately, while it does not harm the ozone
layer, it is a greenhouse gas that has also been implicated in
abnormal testicular growth in rats—so you must have some
serious cojones to keep using it.

Heavy Aromatic Solvent Naphtha

It's not called aromatic because it smells (though it does—like
petroleum). "Aromatic" is a scientific term referring to certain
molecules with one or more hexagonal rings of six carbon
atoms. These molecules can be unusually stable and powerful
solvents for other hydrocarbons. Since naphtha is a mixture of
medium-weight aromatic carbon rings with anywhere from nine

to sixteen carbon atoms (extra carbon atoms can hang off the sides of the main ring structure), this substance easily dissolves smaller carbon compounds like simple plastics but won't harm larger polymers like styrene-butadiene (synthetic tire rubber).

Aromatic Resin

Aromatic hydrocarbon resins are sticky substances made almost exclusively of C_9 monomers (small molecules with nine carbon atoms that can join with other molecules to form polymers). They are commonly used as epoxies and adhesives, and like naphtha and amorphous polyolefin (below), they are found in partially distilled crude oil. Usually all these substances would be further processed and separated, but keeping the resins, naphtha, and polyolefin together works like magic here. How so? Read on.

Amorphous Polyolefin

In the can of Fix-A-Flat, this shapeless mass of polymeric olefins (low-density plastics like polypropylene and polyethylene) remains dissolved in the heavy aromatic naphtha, above. But once Fix-A-Flat is sprayed into the tire, these plastics coat the inner surface of the tire and plug the leak. Then the sticky aromatic resins from above keep the polyolefins in place. The first ingredient, tetrafluoroethane, dries the resins and polyolefins into a stiff rubbery plastic coating, allowing you to drive to the nearest service station to get your tire repaired.

[BACKSTORY]

I never accept freebies for "What's Inside." If I actually need a sample of the item I'm studying, I purchase it at my local supermarket or, in this case, at the auto parts store. I had just finished this piece and went to the library to start researching the next one. I still had the can of Fix-A-Flat in my car when I came out of the library to find I had a flat tire. Not me, actually. My car.

Like many American men (okay, like many *New York* men . . . well, like many New York, lazy, geek, Generation X men), I've never changed a tire before. Maybe I don't drive much or they're making tires better than ever; either way, the situation has never arisen. I wasn't even exactly sure where my jack was.

But the question was moot. I had Fix-A-Flat.

I'm a big believer in reading the instructions before I do something I've never done before. I'm not necessarily a big believer in *following* the instructions, but I like to know

---

GAS

A gas consists of a group of individual atoms or molecules that generally do not touch, like a bunch of people with social anxiety disorder all forced to go to the same party: they'll nervously bounce around the room in a more or less random motion, almost never interacting with each other. And if by chance they bump together, they're more likely to bounce apart than they are to stick together. This differs from a solid, in which the molecules are tightly held together like neurotic codependents, or a liquid, in which the bonds holding the molecules together are so weak they barely stick together, like the narcissistic egomaniacs they are.

what's expected of me. Fix-A-Flat's instructions were very detailed and precise.

First, I had to connect the hose from the can of Fix-A-Flat to the tire's inlet valve. Simple, right? Not to me. I didn't realize that the hose actually screwed onto the valve. I thought it just stuck there.

I hit the trigger, and a high-pressure mixture of fluorocarbons, hydrocarbons, and solute plastics pulsed through the hose. The loose hose disconnected from the tire inlet valve. It whipped around and sprayed me with a combination of aromatic resin and amorphous polyolefin, dissolved in naphtha and propelled by tetrafluoroethane. The bulk of the material landed on my lap.

Fix-A-Flat tells us that when the product is in a liquid state, it can be wiped up with a paper towel, or preferably washed with soap and water. Once it has dried, however, it essentially becomes rubber, and becomes more tenacious: it can only be removed with mineral spirits (a.k.a. the naphtha from which it came), which can be found in hardware stores or art-supply houses. I grabbed some paper towels and sopped up as much of the mess as I could, but already I could feel the edges of the stain start to harden. The end result was that my pants had become impregnated with rapidly solidifying liquid rubber, turning an old pair of jeans into an old pair of jeans with a semiwaterproofed, rubberized crotch area. Eventually the jeans got too old and raggedy to wear, but until the end, the crotch held up amazingly well.

A Flu Shot

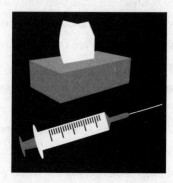

Kills viruses with viruses and ignorance with knowledge.

Hemagglutinin (45 Micrograms)

This is the basis of the vaccine itself. Known as HA, this substance is an antigenic glycoprotein, one of seventeen found in different strains of the influenza virus. HA on a flu virus unlocks your cell membranes—usually in your respiratory system—and gets the bug directly inside your cells, where it can multiply and make you sick. When just HA (without the rest of the virus) is injected into your arm, your immune system can go to work creating hemagglutinin antibodies *without running the risk of getting sick with the flu.*

Sodium Chloride (4.1 Milligrams)

Table salt. Antivaccine advocates want to eliminate this material, which they call a "known mutagen," from vaccines, and, one can only assume, from the rest of our lives as well—why eliminate a mutagen from only one part of your life? That's going to be more than a bit difficult; we need a reasonable amount of table salt to survive. Sure, most people in the developed world take in too much salt each day, but that hasn't mutated them into zombies. Yet.

Ovalbumin (Less Than 1 Microgram)

Egg whites! It starts with a hen and a rooster, inside a henhouse that meets biosecurity requirements for making vaccines. ("Biosecure" means that the birds are protected from outside infection; after all, it's a fool's errand to make human flu vaccine from birds that might be contaminated with avian influenza.) Their fertilized eggs are injected with "seed viruses"—samples of one of this year's expected flu strains. After several days' incubation, the virus-laden egg whites are harvested, purified, and mixed with other flu strains.

Polymyxin B (Less Than 0.5 Nanograms)

An antibacterial compound. It kills germs by altering the permeability of a bacterium's outer membrane, which develops "cracks" that let in hydrophobic compounds, thus killing the cell. It was originally added into the egg that grew the flu viruses, because, let's face it, eggs can be pretty filthy things, and you don't want any bacterial contamination to spoil your virus culture. Have no fear; the FDA is sure that the small amount of polymyxin B that does get through is not likely to cause any severe allergic reactions.

Neomycin Sulfate (Less Than 3 Nanograms)

This is an antibiotic that works by inhibiting the decoding and translocation of RNA inside bacterial cells; the cell's internal mechanism malfunctions, even to the extent of creating abnormal proteins, and the cell dies. Like polymyxin B, it's here to keep the vaccine uncontaminated by bacteria. Too bad it doesn't just limit itself to bacteria, though: neomycin concentrates in the inner-ear fluids of humans, sometimes causing profound hearing loss under the right conditions, like when it is applied directly to ruptured eardrums.

Beta-Propiolactone (Less Than 2 Nanograms)

The virus killer. Perhaps "kill" isn't quite the right word, since viruses aren't exactly alive to begin with. But this stuff "inactivates" the influenza virus, just enough to make it impossible for you to be infected with the flu, but not enough to make it impossible to use in a vaccine. Unfortunately, despite decades of large-scale use of these vaccines, nobody is sure *exactly* how it inactivates a virus and what chemical modifications occur during viral inactivation. Researchers are sure that beta-prop modifies the virus's DNA or RNA. That's a good thing if it happens to a bad virus, but it could be a bad thing if it happens to a healthy cell. This is probably why the International Agency for Research on Cancer (IARC) has classified beta-propiolactone as a Group 2B, possible human carcinogen.

Sodium Taurodeoxycholate (Less Than 10 Parts per Million)

Wicked expensive, with one hundred grams selling for about $3,000. The manufacturer calls this a "bile salt-related, anionic detergent used for isolation of membrane proteins including inner mitochondrial membrane proteins." We call it a virus disruptor. Flu viruses may be inactivated by beta-propiolactone, but they're literally broken apart by this stuff.

[BACKSTORY]

While I was researching this story, I found myself becoming obsessed with actor and comedian Jim Carrey.

In 2007, actress Jenny McCarthy announced that her son had autism, which she claims developed not long after he received a vaccination. McCarthy and Carrey were a couple then, and if you look at photos from any of her antivaccination rallies, you'll see Carrey standing there in the background, holding up a sign questioning the validity of vaccination.

From the expression on his face, it's very reasonable to believe that he wanted to be almost anywhere else. It's hard to know what was going through the poor man's mind: Did he truly believe in the horrors of vaccination? Was he being supportive, joining in with his partner's activities? Or was he just trying to retain Jenny McCarthy?

As I continued to research vaccines, I became convinced that the last reason is the only one that makes any sense, because there is absolutely no scientific basis for McCarthy's antivaccination beliefs. Flu vaccines are, and have been repeatedly proven to be, perfectly safe. *Period.* Of course it's sad that McCarthy's son has whatever neurological disorder he has, but there's no proof that it was caused by vaccines. And it's even sadder that, because McCarthy is a popular figure, thousands, possibly hundreds of thousands, of children around the world are not getting vaccinated. As I write this, there's a measles epidemic raging in New York City, caused entirely by parents who refuse to get their children vaccinated, almost certainly because they feel empowered by McCarthy's uninformed stance.

But, you may say, what's this about the mutagenic effects of sodium chloride? We could find only one study, published in 1987, that explained how much salt you'd need to make a mutant, and they were using yeast cells, not human cells or anything. According to this study, it takes the equivalent of 58.5 milligrams in one injection (about four times as salty as seawater) to make mutated yeast. No idea how to make mutated people, but even if humans mutate as easily as yeast, you'd need fourteen flu shots one right after the other to even stand a chance of mutating yourself with salt.

As for egg white, manufacturers try to separate all the egg white from the virus load, but some always gets through. Don't worry if you have an egg allergy; the amount of ovalbumin in a flu shot is usually too tiny to cause a reaction. If you really can't handle eggs, you can always get a newer flu vaccine that's grown not in chicken eggs but on insect body parts. Ew.

And I admit that the neomycin gives one pause: it would suck to go deaf from a flu shot. Fortunately, that's not going to happen. It would take the neomycin from 580,000 flu shots to equal the amount that is known to harm the ear. That's the equivalent of having 140 two-liter bottles full of flu vaccine injected into you at once. If you do that, you really are just looking for trouble.

Gasoline

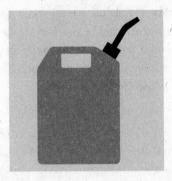

The go juice of our global civilization, in seven easy steps.

Ethyl Tertiary-Butyl Ether

Most of the compounds in gasoline are pure hydrocarbons—molecules that are made of nothing but hydrogen and carbon. But ETBE is not a hydrocarbon. It's an oxygenate—an ingredient that adds more O_2 to the mix. More oxygen helps the fuel to burn steadily into CO_2, carbon dioxide, which is less toxic to humans than carbon monoxide.

Toluene

A derivative of benzene, this pure hydrocarbon is the rootstock of TNT (the official name of which is trinitrotoluene) and is one of the flammable ingredients in gasoline. Inhaling it will get you high, but there is also plenty of evidence that toluene damages your brain. And really, if you're huffing gasoline, you don't need to be any stupider.

Ethanol

Good ol' grain alcohol. It's not found in every blend of gasoline, but when it is, it is used as an oxygenate, much like ETBE, and for the same reasons.

Methyl Tertiary-Butyl Ether

A mixture of methanol (a.k.a. wood alcohol) and isobutylene, MTBE adds oxygen and boosts octane (which means it helps control the burn rate in your car's engine). It was one of several substances that replaced lead in gas. But this additive tends to seep into groundwater, and it is not something you should be drinking, so while it can still be used in much of Asia, its use is being phased out in the United States.

Hexane

Picture it: You're walking through a vibrant neighborhood, one loaded with locally owned shops. There's a butcher's shop. A used bookstore. And over there, in what is usually the smallest store on the block, is a cobbler, someone who makes and repairs shoes. You walk in, and it hits you: that tangy smell you get nowhere else but in an old-fashioned cobbler's shop. It's hexane. Another volatile hydrocarbon, hexane is used as a solvent in shoe glues. It's also used in food factories as a solvent in the extraction of vegetable oils from soybeans and other crops. Yum.

Heptane

In gasoline, heptane is yet another flammable hydrocarbon, but it is more of a contaminant than an ingredient. It is unwelcome in gasoline, because heptane burns explosively—too much heptane in your tank causes the fuel to ignite early and the engine to knock. The stuff is so volatile that flowing heptane can explode from its own built-up static electricity—no external ignition source needed.

Ethylbenzene

Remember the smell of the cobbler's shop a few items back? Walk a bit farther through town until you come to the gas station. That unique smell of gasoline? It's the smell of ethylbenzene, a flammable hydrocarbon. But don't breathe too much of it: it causes birth defects in animals and will ruin your life if it gets in your eyes.

Naphthalene
Use your imagination one more time. You know the scent of naphthalene—it's the characteristic smell of mothballs. Yet another hydrocarbon, naphthalene happens to be lethal to insect larvae, which is why people compress it into little balls and stick them in closets next to their wool suits.

Butane
Yup, the juice in cigarette lighters. A highly versatile chemical feedstock, butane is a building block for many plastics as well as a solvent and, obviously, a fuel.

Pentane
This is the most volatile room-temperature liquid hydrocarbon found in crude oil, helping give gas its explosive power. It is also commonly used in the laboratory as a quick-drying solvent.

Benzene
So important to the mix that in some Slavic languages, the word for gasoline is "benzin." An organic yet carcinogenic hydrocarbon found naturally in petroleum, benzene is just a little too dangerous to keep using—the US government has pledged to cut the use of benzene in gasoline by 45 percent by the year 2030.

[BACKSTORY]

You have to wonder: if gasoline were invented today, would it ever be allowed to be sold to the public? Nearly every ingredient in it is a known harmful substance—benzene is even a listed carcinogen. If gasoline were not grandfathered in, would the EPA and other government agencies ever let the general public handle gasoline without first putting on hazmat equipment? Would they allow giant tanks of the stuff to be stored underground in residential neighborhoods?

One thing we do know—when it comes to being hazardous, modern gasoline is nowhere near as bad as gasoline used to be. In the early 1920s, when the automobile/gasoline industries were finding their footing, they found they had to deal with the annoying problem of engine "knocking." In an

CARBON

This element is *the* fundamental building block of life on Earth, possibly because it is so versatile. To date, scientists have isolated more than ten million known carbon compounds, more than any other element. One reason for this versatility might be carbon's ability to create double bonds with other atoms—bonds that involve four electrons instead of the usual two. Double bonds are unusually strong—perfect for the rough-and-tumble world of living systems. But these bonds are also highly reactive—perfect for the nonstop chemical activity of living systems. With the addition of hydrogen, carbon is the basis of petroleum and plastics. Carbon, hydrogen, and oxygen are the basis of fats, sugars, and alcohols. Add nitrogen and sulfur to that group and you've got amino acids and proteins. Add phosphorus and you've got the building blocks of DNA and RNA. And none of these would be possible without carbon.

internal combustion engine, knocking occurs when the engine's fuel-air mixture explodes prematurely, or too late, or any time it's not supposed to. In the early 1920s, two General Motors researchers, Thomas Midgley and Charles Kettering, discovered that they could minimize and even eliminate engine knocking by adding a small percentage of a compound known as tetraethyl lead to gasoline.

You can think of tetraethyl lead as a single atom of lead surrounded by four ethyl (CH_3) molecules. As the gasoline burns inside an internal combustion engine, that tetraethyl lead is converted to lead oxide, which actually slows down the combustion and makes the gasoline burn more smoothly, thus eliminating nearly all engine knocking.

Of course all this lead bouncing around the engine didn't do the engine much good, because the lead oxide had a tendency to deposit in the fuel system, leading to a kind of heavy metal sclerosis of the engine. In order to protect car engines from this problem, researchers quickly learned to add another chemical, dibromoethane, to the fuel. Dibromoethane, which is made of two molecules of bromine and a hydrocarbon, combines with the lead in the car's cylinders. The resulting bromine-lead compound simply vaporizes out of the expensive, valuable car engine and into the atmosphere, which is free.

The problem was that even back then, scientists knew lead was a health problem. The advertising teams who marketed this gasoline simply called it "ethyl," leaving out all mention of lead, in the time-honored tradition of "What the public doesn't know won't be traced back to us. We hope." (You'll occasionally hear characters in movies from the thirties and forties talking about buying "ethyl" when they stop at a gas station.)

But the researchers, especially Midgley, knew the problem with lead was real; just like the Mad Hatter in *Alice in Wonderland* (hatmakers of Victorian times were especially prone to heavy-metal poisoning from the mercury they used to make felt), many of the researchers working on leaded gasoline routinely suffered from lung problems, cognitive deficiencies, hallucinations, and insanity. After Midgley's second bout of lead poisoning, which required a year's convalescence in Europe, he was taken off leaded gasoline research and transferred to another department at GM.

This new department, located in the frigid-air section of General Motors, was dedicated to finding a safe refrigerator fluid. In those days, refrigerator coils were commonly filled with volatile gases like ammonia. A leak from a faulty refrigerator could, and frequently did, asphyxiate whole families. In fact, one of Albert Einstein's inventions (did you know he was an inventor?) was a refrigerator that did not use poisonous ammonia gas.

Midgley, perhaps as penance, worked strenuously to develop a new, safe form of refrigerant. His goal was to find a compound that was volatile enough to use as a refrigerant yet completely chemically inert. By 1930, he and his team were producing the first commercially viable chlorofluorocarbon, which he named Freon. At last Midgley had his redemption for introducing lead into the atmosphere—he had invented a gas that was totally nonreactive. Totally harmless.

Midgley died, severely disabled, in 1944 at age fifty-five. Not long after, researchers began to realize that Midgley's Freon wasn't as nonreactive or as harmless as he had thought. Once Freon and other chlorofluorocarbons migrated up into the stratosphere, unfiltered ultraviolet light broke apart the Freon molecules. The result was a highly reactive chlorine ion, floating around the stratosphere voraciously looking for something to bond with. Such as a molecule of ozone.

Ozone is the name for triatomic oxygen (O_3), that is, a molecule made of three oxygen atoms. Ozone has a pretty interesting property that relates to life on Earth: the particular structure of three oxygen atoms very efficiently absorbs ultraviolet light. When an ozone molecule is hit by an ultraviolet ray, it splits apart into an oxygen molecule (O_2) and a single atom of oxygen. The atomic oxygen almost immediately recombines with an O_2 molecule to re-create ozone. If left to itself, this process can go on forever; ultraviolet light gets absorbed in the stratosphere, so it is unlikely to harm living creatures on Earth's surface, while the ozone molecules that do the absorbing are continuously created, destroyed, and re-created again.

The addition of Freon, and its payload of chlorine atoms, changes all of that. Now, when an ozone molecule is broken apart by an ultraviolet ray, the unpaired oxygen atom can meet up with a chlorine atom to create chlorine monoxide (ClO). This leaves behind an O_2 molecule in the stratosphere, and O_2 is not very good at absorbing ultraviolet rays. If that chlorine monoxide molecule meets up with another ozone molecule, it can destroy that ozone molecule as well, leaving behind two molecules of oxygen and an unattached chlorine atom, which starts the cycle all over again. In this process, ozone gets destroyed by Freon and not rebuilt.

It would be thirty years before the ozone-depleting effects of Midgley's chlorofluorocarbons would become known and words like "ozone hole" entered the public's consciousness.

184

At roughly the same time, Midgley's lead was being phased out of gasoline for being an environmental hazard.

For his contributions to the environment, Georgetown University professor J. R. McNeill said that Midgley "had more impact on the atmosphere than any other single organism in Earth's history."

Head & Shoulders Shampoo

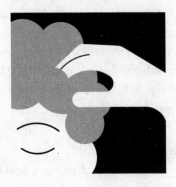

Use anything, just get rid of this yeast infection on my scalp!

Pyrithione Zinc

Dandruff is caused by a yeast infection. Yeast eats your scalp secretions and metabolizes them into oleic acid. Oleic acid in turn attacks the membranes of your skin cells, which causes an increase in cell production, and thus an increase in dead skin cells. These dead skin cells turn into dry white flakes that fall on your shoulders (though only if you are predisposed to dandruff—some people don't react to oleic acid). Pyrithione zinc depolarizes yeast cell membranes, which is like locking all the doors and windows into the cell. Your scalp citizens will soon find themselves unable to ingest secretions or excrete waste, and they will quickly die.

Polyquaternium-10

For something with a name like a sci-fi planet, this ingredient is pretty humdrum. It's a moisturizer (it helps provide the "dry scalp care") and an antistatic agent (now that your pate is free of dead skin, you don't need to look like a live wire).

Zinc Carbonate

A bright blue mineral (which helps to explain why so many dandruff shampoos are blue). Formerly called calamine (as in lotion) and now called smithsonite (after the man whose money was used to found the Smithsonian), this astringent was used in the old days to dry up skin lesions (such as those caused by seborrhoeic dermatitis, or severe dandruff) that might have weepy, moist discharges. Here, it also ensures that the pyrithione stays mixed and effective.

Sodium Laureth Sulfate

Though the yeast may be killed, their oleic acid remains behind. This is a detergent and foaming agent common in shampoos; the detergent lifts grease and dirt off your scalp and hair, but the foam is cosmetic—people just like foamy cleansers.

Dimethicone

There is natural oil on your hair, and when you wash it all away, your follicles are clean, dry ... and unprotected. Dimethicone is a silicone-based oil—you might know it as the squishy stuff inside breast implants—that conditions and protects the hair until its natural oils build up again.

Glycol Distearate

This waxy substance adds a milky pearlescent quality to the shampoo. It does nothing to clean hair, but it is psychologically vital: according to Head & Shoulders maker Procter & Gamble, opaque shampoos are perceived by the public as gentle. Since dandruff shampoo is by necessity a pourable killing machine you put on your head, you want some reassurance that everything will turn out all right in the end.

Magnesium Sulfate and Magnesium Carbonate Hydroxide

P & G tells us that these are excipients, substances that help the active ingredient, pyrithione zinc, work more effectively. In this instance, the excipients probably work to lower the surface tension of the water in the shampoo, to keep the pyrithione zinc well suspended in the solution and encourage it to home in on your scalp.

Methylchloroisothiazolinone and Methylisothiazolinone

These two preservatives kill any bacteria that form in the bottle. In a test tube, methylisothiazolinone (MIT) has been proven to kill neurons, but don't worry: even the European Union, which is generally much stricter than the FDA, agrees that MIT is safe in shampoo. So that should be a weight off your shoulders.

Blue Dye #1

Okay, so maybe the zinc carbonate isn't *quite* enough to make the shampoo blue.

DANDRUFF

So many of our great diseases—Tourette's, Alzheimer's, Parkinson's—are named after the doctor who first described them or first characterized the symptoms as a disease. It's one of the compensations for the low pay and hard work of a research scientist; you get to name your discoveries after yourself.

When Louis-Charles Malassez was a young medical student in Paris in 1867, he no doubt had such dreams. Perhaps he had already heard of the pioneering, lifesaving work Louis Pasteur was doing in the field of immunology. Perhaps he had heard of Ignaz Semmelweis's work on reducing the spread of disease by having doctors simply wash their hands between patients. Malassez probably sat and wondered what his research destiny held, what great disease would bear his name.

When the Germans invaded France in 1870, Malassez joined the Fifth Ambulance Corps as a field medic. The intense on-the-job training he received in battle led to his receiving the chair of anatomy at the Collège de France in 1875. Was it then that his career took off? Certainly, he made a name for himself studying blood cells, and also did some pioneering work in the field of dentistry. But those accomplishments are pretty well forgotten. What is Louis-Charles Malassez's most enduring claim to fame?

He isolated and described a particularly disgusting genus of fungi, specifically the species *Malassezia globosa*, the skin fungus that causes dandruff.

Heroin

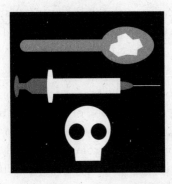

Whatchoo gonna do with all that junk?

Diacetylmorphine

This chemical is the real stuff: pharmaceutical-grade heroin. Marketed by Bayer as an over-the-counter cough suppressant in 1898, it's fairly easy to make out of raw opium, some chemicals, and basic lab equipment. The percentage of diacetylmorphine in street heroin can vary based on geographic source; South American wholesale has been falling from a high of 88 percent in 2003. Street purity in the US has been around 35 percent in recent years.

Caffeine

When added in the lab while the heroin is still in solution, this results in hard thumbnail-sized "crystals" of heroin, which can be smoked like crack. If you add it to processed, powdered heroin, the mixture will vaporize at a lower temperature, making it easier to "chase the dragon": to inhale heroin vapors through a straw.

Noscapine

Heroin got its name from the German word "*heroisch*," meaning "heroic," perhaps because of its *heroisch* ability to suppress coughs. The opium by-product noscapine may also help: it's believed to act on the body's sigma receptors, which can regulate the cough reflex. Noscapine is also being looked at for its promising anticancer powers. Perhaps this stuff is the reason Keith Richards is still with us?

Mannitol

This is a sugar alcohol that increases osmotic pressure in the intestines, making it a gentle and effective laxative. Since heroin is a wicked constipator (seriously slowing down the intestines), is the mannitol a thoughtful gift from your friendly neighborhood dealer? Hardly. Adding any white, powdery stuff to heroin lets him sell less drug for the same amount of money.

Monoacetylmorphine

Heroin's technical name is diacetylmorphine: two acetyl groups connected to a morphine molecule. This is morphine with just one acetyl group. The average bag of street heroin contains quite a bit of this stuff, and even more is made inside of you: brain enzymes break off one of the heroin's acetyl groups, leaving this form, which is actually more potent than heroin but harder to extract in the lab. Back in the 1990s, a lot of drug-testing kits would respond to just about any poppy-based compound, leading to the possibility that eating a poppy-seed bagel would yield a positive result. Nowadays, more and more drug tests actually search for this specific compound, which is not found in a bagel and is solid evidence of heroin use.

Acetaminophen

A key ingredient in Percocet and several migraine remedies but a potentially lethal adulterant in high doses. Heroin cut with acetaminophen is often sold on the street as "cheese."

Papaverine

Raw opium is a goulash of many different compounds; badly processed street skag can retain many of them. This poppy alkaloid is useless to junkies because it won't make them high, but it does have legitimate medical use as a vasodilator that relaxes smooth muscle, thereby increasing blood flow. Imagine, a heroin by-product that helps people survive a stroke.

Quinine

Junkie lore says that dealers added this to the supply as a public service, after a malaria outbreak among needle-sharing users in the 1930s. Still found in low-quality junk, it has a bitter taste that mimics heroin's bite (caveat emptor) and supposedly adds to the rush. But quinine is bad stuff to be injecting—it can cause blindness and has been a key factor in some heroin ODs.

Dextromethorphan

This cough syrup mainstay is known to reduce some effects of heroin detox (runny nose, twitching, insomnia). But a dealer's job is not to make withdrawal easier; DXM may be here for its pharmacological effects—hallucinations and euphoria. Unwelcome bonus: at high doses, it can induce psychosis.

[BACKSTORY]

O h, man.

Oh, man!

This one was bad.

I visited the first place in North America where heroin was sold (sold legally, I might add!); the address is now an Italian restaurant in a part of New York City's Hanover Square that has been kept from development. I didn't expect to see anything—I just wanted a feel for the place where our heroin mess more or less began.

I interviewed an old junkie (yes, some of them do make it to old age) and read old-junkie memoirs.

I tried to interview people from Bayer (the first marketers of heroin, back when it was legal), but they wanted nothing to do with my story. I visited medical libraries and I visited hospitals.

And I feel as though I read every single blog kept by people trying to get themselves off of heroin or trying to get a loved one off heroin. And each new piece of data got me more

---

CHEMICAL REACTIONS

The International Union of Pure and Applied Chemistry defines a chemical reaction as "a process that leads to the transformation of one set of chemical substances to another." This simple sentence is essentially the software for life, which at its most basic is nothing but a series of chemical reactions. The four basic reactions are *synthesis* (e.g., hydrogen and oxygen coming together to make water), *decomposition* (e.g., table sugar breaking apart into glucose and fructose), *single replacement* (e.g., silver nitrate combined with pure zinc producing zinc nitrate and pure silver), and *double replacement* (e.g., acetic acid and sodium bicarbonate producing sodium acetate, carbon dioxide, and water).

and more upset and depressed. There are few things as insidiously evil as heroin.

When I first decided to find out what was inside heroin, I was excited about looking into this powder that was powerful enough to make someone throw their life away.

People around me were more wary of this story. My girlfriend laid down some rules: you're not buying any heroin, she said, and if you do buy any you're *not* bringing it into the house, and you are definitely not using heroin in any way. My editors were equally uneasy. Don't do anything stupid, was their advice. It's simultaneously flattering and disquieting to know that people around me think I am gonzo enough to go out and score smack, let alone use it! To tell the truth, before I started researching the story, I didn't even have any idea where to buy the stuff.

On the lighter side: the photo editor contacted me and said they didn't want to photograph a mountain of baby powder and call it heroin. We wanted the real stuff. Our photographer was in England at the time, so I called Scotland Yard and got their narcotics division. I asked if we could send a photographer and art director into their evidence room, break open a kilo of China White, and take some pictures. The officer I spoke to was very nice, but she said that as much as they liked the idea of the article, the Metropolitan Police were under intense public/governmental scrutiny as to how they allocated their resources, and it was not in their best interests to devote a couple of officers to spending all day monitoring a photo shoot that wouldn't appear in the UK anyway. Then—and I'm sure she didn't mean it as an insult—she said, "The US is awash in heroin. Wouldn't it be easier to shoot your pictures there?"

So, what did we actually end up using in the photograph? I'll tell you when the statute of limitations runs out.

This Is What You Put on Your Head

Just For Men Hair Color

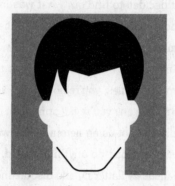

There ain't no words for the beauty, the splendor, the monochrome chemical eyesore of my hair. . . .

Ethoxydiglycol

Back in the 1930s, home hair dyes were laced with toxic chemicals that turned a simple touch-up into a hazmat adventure. Luckily, dye makers found substitutes like EDG, a fume-free organic solvent that keeps the ingredients in a thin, pourable consistency until needed.

Oleyl Alcohol, Vegetable Fatty Acid

However, keeping the ingredients in a thin, pourable consistency would be a problem when you're trying to apply the dye. These two fatty organic thickeners kick in when you mix the dye base with the separate bottle of "color developer," making the product cling to your hair like shampoo.

Ethanolamine

This is one of the key solvents in Easy-Off oven cleaner. With the properties of an alcohol (ethanol) and ammonia (amine), this single chemical can do the job of both. The alcohol side removes excess water from hair, keeping the dye from being diluted. The amine side boosts the pH toward bleachlike levels and swells the hair's outer layer, so the color can penetrate more fully.

Erythorbic Acid

If you take ascorbic acid—a.k.a. vitamin C—and rearrange the atoms just so (a process we like to call isomerization), you get erythorbic acid. It's a cheap antioxidant without any of its cousin's vitamin properties. Since biological colors can be damaged with exposure to sunlight and oxygen, an antioxidant is a good thing if you're going to lie about your hair.

Trisodium EDTA

With its ability to bind heavy metals, EDTA is used to clean up after radioactive spills. That same talent is enlisted here to suck up copper in tap water, which might otherwise react with the product to create radicals that could damage your hair proteins; dyed hair is messed up enough already.

Polyquaternium-22

Sounds like a chemical from the golden age of comic books, but in reality, it's just four amine groups attached to a nitrogen atom. This common polymer coats each strand of hair, smoothing the shaft's outer layer and improving lubricity—a fancy way of saying it's a hair conditioner.

p-Aminophenol, p-Phenylenediamine Sulfate

These so-called intermediates react inside the hair fiber (which has been opened up by the ethanolamine, if you remember) to produce the appropriate color when oxidized. This combination, heavy in sulfur, turns dark brown. Other chemicals (or different proportions of these) can make any natural hair shade—from Sandy Blond to Jet Black.

Resorcinol

Is there anything this stuff can't do? It's used as a chemical skin peel, a biological glue for aortic surgery, a sunscreen, a treatment for whooping cough, and—when mixed with the right acids—a TNT-like explosive. In Just For Men, it's a coupler, an additive that reacts with the oxidized intermediates to dial in the target color.

Hydrogen Peroxide

When combined with the other ingredients, this ubiquitous denizen of the medicine cabinet provides a superabundance of highly reactive oxygen, which turns those intermediates and couplers into luxurious dark coloring that will surely fool everyone (and possibly even yourself) into thinking that if your hair looks young, you must also look young.

[BACKSTORY]

Like a good journalist, I felt it was necessary to test the product thoroughly before writing about it.

Ever since my hair started going gray while I was being tortured by the federal government (no, I wasn't in Guantanamo; I worked at the Federal Reserve Bank of New York, which is the next worst thing), I had half-joked about dying my hair red. Bright red. Clown red. *Run Lola Run* red. Over the years, the idea and the tint has faded; I was willing to settle for a slightly more biologically reasonable deep orange color, the carotene color of natural "red" hair. But still, for various reasons that added up to no real reason at all, I never colored my hair.

But now I had a reason. I was doing it for science! When it came time to start work on this article, I bought a box of Just For Men Sandy Blond hair color (they don't make a red hair mix, and Sandy Blond came closest to what I wanted). On a hot Friday night I started the forty-eight-hour allergen test, as recommended on the box, to see if this stuff would send me into anaphylactic shock.

OXIDATION

Originally, oxidation was seen simply as the addition of an oxygen atom to a particular molecule to form an oxide. Often this happens under high heat or burning: flaming hydrogen joins with oxygen to form H_2O, which is technically dihydrogen oxide. Heated nitrogen will combine with oxygen to form nitric oxide. Under less energetic conditions, iron will slowly combine with oxygen to form rust, or ferric oxide. As scientists came to understand the process better, they realized that oxygen is not necessary; the process of oxidation really is based around the loss of electrons.

As it says on the Just For Men website: "Just For Men has a new True Color Formula that targets only the gray hair—replaces it with subtle tones that match your own natural color." Remember those words.

My natural hair is a kind of dark dusty brown. There is one huge patch of gray, about the size of an outstretched palm, on my right temporal zone above my ear. There are other gray hairs scattered throughout the rest of my head like milkweeds in a field of barley. Since Just For Men targets "only the gray," my idea was to leave my dusty brown hair dusty brown but color the gray Sandy Blond so that I would have dusty brown hair with Sandy Blond highlights scattered throughout seemingly at random (with the obvious exception of a huge Sandy Blond patch on the right temporal lobe, which I could live with). I honestly believed this would happen.

On Sunday night I snapped on the gloves, mixed and shook the bottles, then glopped the warm, chemically reacting mixture onto my hair. As the instructions suggested, I started with the area that was most gray, then worked to the rest of my head. The instructions said to leave the hair color on for five minutes to reach the desired shade—leaving it on for a longer time results in a darker color, while a shorter time might not "take." I waited exactly five minutes, waited a few seconds more, then stepped into the shower.

As the water poured down on me, great gobs of brown goo came off my head and dirtied the bathtub. My first reaction was that this was Not Good. The instructions said to shampoo, so I shampooed my hair until the lather and water ran clear.

I stepped out of the shower, looked into the mirror, and

did not recognize the creature peering back at me. Just For Men may indeed target only the gray, but the rest of my hair was an unintended casualty: the dye had colored all my hair, not just the gray. My head was now monochrome, a sight I hadn't seen since the days of acid-washed jeans: a glossy milk-chocolatey brown that I've never had in my life, and should not have come out of this product! And I started having a major existential freak-out. There appears to be something about coloring one's hair that can lead to serious thoughts in the *Who am I, what am I doing?* vein.

The fascinating thing is that no one else had any problem with my new hair color. In fact, based on the reactions I got over the next few days, I don't think anyone even noticed. No one asked if I had changed my hair. No one commented on my new youthful appearance. No one even said, "Hmm, there's something different about you but I can't put my finger on it." Nada. Nothing. I eventually spent most of one afternoon shampooing—lather, rinse, repeat in an endless loop—until I had washed the gray back into my hair.

This Is What You Put on Your Special Area

K-Y Yours+Mine Couples Lubricants

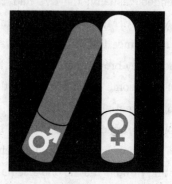

Also known as the adventures of the sugar stick and the vale of tears.

BOTH:
Propylene Glycol

Yes, yes, yes, you're spreading brake fluid on your special region. But it's the good kind of brake fluid: practically nontoxic (well, very low toxicity) and recognized as food safe by the FDA. But put the brakes on overusing it, as it's also recognized as a possible vaginal irritant in some women (i.e., those with vulvodynia—chronic pain, burning, or irritation in the area around the opening of the vagina).

. . . .

HERS:
Menthyl Lactate

Described by chemists as "faintly minty in odor and virtually tasteless with a pleasant, long-lasting cooling effect," menthyl lactate triggers the TRPM8 receptors in the skin, creating a psychophysical sensation of cold (this is probably what K-Y calls "tingling") without actually lowering the skin's temperature. Which makes sense, because a cold shower is the last thing you need if you're using this stuff.

. . . .

Methyl Salicylate

Wintergreen oil, which produces a warm, almost burning sensation, possibly by activating the skin's TRPA1 pain receptors as well as the ANKTM1 receptors, which seems to activate multiple cold and pain signals (really, the science of these things is all over the place). By combining these two ingredients, you're essentially coating the Feminine Mystery with a layer of Icy Hot. Hot and tingly might be just how you want to be on V-Day, but be careful; this stuff can cause temporary numbness and swelling of the tongue.

Hydroxyethylcellulose

The human body, amazing machine though it is, is also a lazy sod that reuses anything it can. That's why tears, mucus, saliva, and natural vaginal lubrication are all so similar—they're all made from the same basic ingredients in different proportions. So when it comes time to whip up a batch of artificial *jus d'amour*, where else to go but the stuff used in some artificial tears? This can be made from wood or cotton, and it's just about perfect for the job: it can be formulated to come out of the container heavy and rich and then thin out, feeling wet and dispersing easily on the flesh.

Benzoic Acid

The K-Y people were presented with a problem: how to prevent mold and bacteria from growing in this soup of natural oils and food-safe ingredients, without harming the person who is going to apply this to their mucous membranes. They opted for benzoic acid, which kills yeasts by messing with their ATP molecules, the "batteries" of living cells. Benzoic acid works best when pH is below 4.5, and luckily, natural vaginal pH is ideally between 3.5 and 4.5.

Sodium Hydroxide

The great Renaissance physician Paracelsus is famous for his adage "All things are poison, and nothing is without poison; only the dose permits something not to be poisonous." You'd better hope he's right; this is lye, and you're spreading it on your Special Area. Actually, it's here to regulate the pH of the product—remember the problem with benzoic acid and vaginal pH—and the dose is tiny enough to be harmless.

. . . .

HIS:
Honey

The stickiest food in the known universe doesn't seem to fit with the slip-'n'-slide nature of the product. Plus, is it wise to put honey inside your honey? K-Y says its formulation is perfectly safe, which is more than most people can say about love.

. . . .

Glycerin

This sweet, odorless, colorless, oily, viscous liquid is a chemical for all seasons. In various products it's used as an emulsifier, a moisturizer, a solvent, an antifreeze, and (with the addition of nitrogen) an explosive. It's found in suppositories, syrups, and soaps. As a sweetener, it's got 1.08 times the calories of sugar. Oh, and it's also very, very slippery, making it perfect for the job of love grease.

. . . .

Maltodextrin

Did you ever wonder what the difference between "Sugars" and "Total Carbohydrates" on a food label is? This stuff makes up part of that difference. A collection of glucose molecules from either cornstarch, rice starch, potato starch, or tapioca, maltodextrin can be used as a mild sweetener in its own right, though it's more commonly just used as a filler. As a pharmaceutical excipient, maltodextrin can help with increasing a solution's viscosity, to prevent the crystallization of syrups or to create films such as on tablet coatings (though that's unlikely here).

Sucralose

This is Splenda, the artificial sweetener in the bright yellow packets, so intensely sugary that it is usually cut with maltodextrin (above) to keep it from being too cloying. Are you noticing a trend? *Every single ingredient in the "for him" lubricant is edible and sweet.* Aside from turning the penis into a lollipop, do you think the K-Y people are surreptitiously providing a critique of the rewards of sex and gender in postmodern society? Or is it just an accident that the man gets the honey and the woman gets artificial tears?

This Is What You Put on Your Face

Neutrogena Healthy Skin
Face Lotion SPF 15

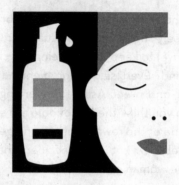

A nongreasy blend of face-melting acids, diesel exhaust, and vitamins.

Hydroxyacetic Acid

Marketers prefer the less-scary-sounding "alpha-hydroxy." It's a corrosive acid that breaks apart the outer layer of skin, spurring new cell growth. While it may make you look younger, it can also make skin twice as vulnerable to sun damage—good thing Neutrogena adds SPF 15 sunscreen. When hydroxyacetic acid is not melting faces worldwide, it can be found in bathroom tile scum removers, where it dissolves minerals left behind in your shower.

. . . .

Benzoic Acid

A derivative of toluene and oxygen, benzoic acid is a preservative commonly used to keep soda or fruit juice from getting moldy. In lotion, it functions as an antimicrobial.

. . . .

Benzophenone

Rub this flower-scented lotion on your skin or stick your face in a diesel's tailpipe, where benzophenone is present in the exhaust. Either way, you get a nice sunscreen. If swallowed or inhaled, though, the substance may disrupt hormones and mess with your brain. Scientists—and probably industry lawyers—recommend against using it on kids.

Panthenol
This is the alcohol variant of pantothenic acid, a.k.a. vitamin B5. In a living cell, it becomes a component of coenzyme A, which helps repair the skin's plasma membranes. Attention Fukushima-area residents: it also protects against gamma radiation from nuclear fallout.

Retinyl Palmitate
The good news is that vitamin A really does help against various skin disorders like acne. The better news: in clinical trials, it has been known to flush out residual leukemia cells that remain after conventional chemotherapy.

Ascorbic Acid Polypeptide
You know it as vitamin C. In lab tests, ascorbic acid generated an eightfold increase in the production of collagen, which helps prevent wrinkles. It's also a powerful antioxidant that neutralizes free radicals (highly reactive molecules that can damage the skin's surface).

Octyl Methoxycinnamate
Another sunscreen ingredient, this compound absorbs light in the 280-to-320-nanometer range, the ultraviolet-B part of the spectrum. This type of blocker is a fairly recent addition to lotions—the ozone layer used to stop UVB rays.

Xanthan Gum
This natural additive gets around more than a sneeze in a subway car. A polysaccharide carefully harvested from huge

vats of *Xanthomonas campestris* bacteria, it provides a smooth, pillowy texture in just about everything—from toothpaste and ice cream to rust dissolver.

SUNSCREEN

As the first protohumans left Africa, they also left behind an easy hunter-gatherer lifestyle, a stable climate, and an intact SLC24A5 gene. This gene, which codes for dark skin color, mutated in these wanderers to lose a single amino acid, which led to most of the coloration difference between Africans and Europeans.

The mutation of SLC24A5 was clearly beneficial for the wanderers: lighter skin absorbs more ultraviolet light, which interacts with molecules of 7-dehydrocholesterol in the skin and turns them into molecules of vitamin D, allowing the migrating groups to populate higher latitudes that don't get as much UV light through the atmosphere. Without this free source of vitamins, humans would have to work harder to obtain foods rich in vitamin D.

But the mutation of SLC24A5 was also clearly detrimental to the wanderers: lighter skin absorbs more ultraviolet light, which is so energetic it can rip apart the DNA of skin cells, leading to various types of cancer.

Human ingenuity thought it was up to the task. Ancient Greeks and Romans coated themselves with a thin layer of olive oil, hoping for protection from the sun. In reality, olive oil does nothing to stop ultraviolet light; at best, it might help to moisturize the skin and repair the damage done by the sun. (And this practice continued until at least the early 1970s with my nana, who herself dated back to ancient Rome, slathering extra-virgin Genco Pura on whichever grandchildren she managed to capture when the family went to the beach.)

Other ancient remedies centered around repairing a sunburn. Egyptians used a poultice of marigold flowers on burned skin. This actually works, since marigolds contain calendula, which is so effective at repairing skin that four thousand years later, doctors give it to patients undergoing radiation therapy, to keep their skin safe.

What we commonly think of as modern-day sunscreen was invented nearly simultaneously by four men in different corners of the globe. Swiss chemistry student Fritz Greiter started working on sunscreen after he got a bad sunburn in the Alps. Florida pharmacist Benjamin Green was a member of a high-altitude airplane crew in World War II and wanted to do something to prevent their high-altitude sunburns. Frenchman Eugene Schueller was the head of cosmetics giant L'Oréal and recognized the need to protect the skin from sun damage, and South Australian chemist Milton Blake needed something to protect his skin in the outback.

All these men focused on the same chemical compounds—ring-shaped molecules that could absorb ultraviolet light without breaking down themselves: the basis of nearly every sunscreen to this day. Together they created an industry worth nearly eleven billion dollars in the US alone, and, more important, one that has saved countless lives.

This Is What You Put on Your Skin

Noxzema

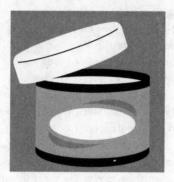

Pig gelatin and plant extracts, and did we mention the pig gelatin?

Stearic Acid

Trivial name for octadecanoic acid, a long-chain, saturated fatty acid, often found in triglycerides, commonly found in tallow, lard, coconuts, and cocoa. You may have a few pounds of this sitting around the house right now, since it is probably the most commonly used fat in soaps, cosmetic creams, and lotions. While pure stearic acid is generally hard to the touch, frequently what's called "stearic acid" in commercial products is actually a mix of different fats, resulting in a waxy solid. Think of it as Vaseline from cows.

. . . .

Linum Usitatissimum Seed Oil (Linseed)

Pressed from the dried, ripe bodies of *Linum usitatissimum* seeds, this oil is used as a nutritional supplement, a putty, and a binder for oil paints. It can dry into a tough plasticlike substance that is the "lin-" in old-fashioned linoleum floors. It can act as a surfactant in cosmetics, but Noxzema specifically says that its moisturizing properties make it useful as a skin conditioner and moisturizer.

. . . .

Glycine Soja Oil (Soybean)

More triglycerides. In your body, too many triglycerides are associated with problems like increased cholesterol and can lead to heart disease. On your skin, however, they're soft, sweet moisturizers.

. . . .

Propylene Glycol

Have you ever heard of contact urticaria? It's a skin condition, commonly known as hives, which presents, the scientists say, as a "hypersensitivity reaction that appears on the skin following contact with an eliciting substance." Such as propylene glycol. While the connection between urticaria and propylene glycol is well established, the FDA still keeps the substance on the Generally Regarded As Safe (GRAS) list. Today, propylene glycol is allowed to be up to 50 percent of a cosmetic product; too bad that some sensitive people can get a reaction at 2 percent.

. . . .

Gelatin

Hydrolyzed pig collagen—that is, the organic material of the bones, the tendons, the cartilage, and the skin of what Unilever delicately calls "pork sources." When mixed with acid and exposed to increasingly hot water, the collagen protein chains are broken apart—"depolymerized" is the cold, scientific term— then dried and ground up for later use. While the inclusion of pork might make Noxzema haram (unfit for use by Muslims), according to at least one kosher certification organization, under the right circumstances it is perfectly permissible for Jewish people to use pork gelatin. Though perhaps not on the Sabbath, when there's a prohibition against smearing or smoothing things like ointments or creams. This leads to the ancient Talmudic question: is Noxzema an ointment or a cream? Do face washes applied and smoothed across the face break the rules? Whatever you do, just don't eat it.

. . . .

Camphor

Noxzema used to be advertised as something that "knocks eczema," a painful skin condition. The active ingredient in mothballs (at least the old-fashioned ones that float), camphor has been used as a drug for centuries: it is rapidly absorbed through the skin and has proven anti-itch qualities, which must have been a great relief for hand scratchers one hundred years ago. These days, parent company Unilever shies away from claims that Noxzema has any curative powers at all, so camphor is probably here for its other effects: it smells nice, and it creates a feeling of coolness on the skin, which can be followed by a local-anesthetic effect.

Ammonium Hydroxide

Ammonia dissolved in water. Since some of the other ingredients like phenol are acidic, the manufacturers are most likely using this strong alkaline substance as a pH balancer to keep the product mild.

Phenol

Phenol was the miracle drug of the nineteenth century: a broad-spectrum antiseptic that made postoperative infection rates plummet. Since raw phenol can be a bit harsh—causing bleaching or numbing of the skin—it's not used much these days as a disinfectant; some formulations of Noxzema leave it out altogether. That might be a bit disconcerting: Noxzema's signature Proustian "library paste" aroma is due to this chemical.

Menthol

What's more natural than Noxzema on a sunburn? Plenty, as it turns out. Noxzema was made back in the days when people put butter on burned skin, which we now know is probably the worst thing you can do—butter can seal in the heat and can lead to infection. A coating of Noxzema might not be any better: the company specifically does not recommend using it on a sunburn. So why does Noxzema feel *so good* on a sunburn? Probably because of this stuff, an extract of Japanese mint that excites the skin's cold-receptor nerves into thinking the temperature has dropped when it hasn't.

[BACKSTORY]

There are so many stories about the history of Noxzema, it's hard to know what's true and what's not. Was it invented in Baltimore by pharmacist George Bunting? Or did Bunting obtain the formula from someone else? Did Noxzema gets its name from a customer who exclaimed, "That stuff really knocked my eczema"? Or was that just a marketing ploy? Maybe none of the stories are true.

As usual, in early July 2013 I purchased a jar of the stuff (my first one in years) to try it out before researching it. Noxzema still has the same library-paste scent that I remembered, but the jar was no longer the heavy cobalt-blue glass of my childhood.

Over the next two weeks, I determined that Noxzema works well as a face wash, a body wash, and a shaving cream. It is not an effective shampoo. It does provide relief to sunburned skin, whether the company wants to admit it or not. I was so happy with it that I really felt that there was going to be room in our lives for more Noxzema. Until the middle of July.

"Hey, look at this," I said to my girlfriend after a particularly juicy bit of research. "A group of Orthodox rabbis have said that it is okay to use pork-based skin products as long as you don't use them on Saturday. Apparently you're not allowed to spread ointment on the Sabbath."

"Who makes pork-based skin products?" she asked.

"Noxzema. It contains gelatin that's pork based."

"Pork?" she asked.

I knew this was trouble. "Well, 'pork sources,'" I admitted.

"*Pork?*" she asked again. "I've been using that on my *face!*"

I still continued to use Noxzema to wash my hands and face. Two days later I developed hard itchy red bumps on my hands, forehead, nose, and jawline.

"What the hell is this?" I said as I scratched the weals.

"I'm no doctor," she said, "but it looks to me like contact urticaria, a skin condition commonly known as hives."

That was our last jar of Noxzema for a while.

This Is What You Put in Your Hands

Play-Doh

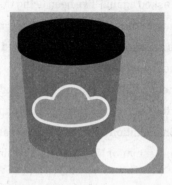

*Simple grains from the earth, simple water from the sky,
simple radiation blocking minerals from Death Valley . . .*

Flour and Water

This is what the other toy manufacturers, with their clays, foams, and silicone-polymer modeling compounds, never seemed to grasp: dough is cheap, and kids love to play with it. The 1965 patent for Play-Doh called for hard winter wheat, which is high in bindy, springy gluten; new Play-Doh formulations allow for wheat, rice, rye, and even tapioca. Celiacs: wash your hands after playing.

Salt

Too much water (or a normal amount of water for a long period of time) could let enzymes go to work on the dough, turning the flour's complex starches into simple sugars and leaving behind nothing but a sweet puddle. Making the dough about 10 percent salt (most bread dough is about 1.5 percent) binds up any excess water.

Amylopectin

Straight-chain starch molecules have an annoying habit of attaching to themselves over time, pushing out water molecules and turning the dough hard and crumbly—we call it going stale. Scientists call this retrogradation. This waxy starch is a retrogradation inhibitor: its branched structure resists clumping by providing hidey-holes for water molecules, keeping Play-Doh moist and pliable.

Mineral or Vegetable Oil
Flour and water (and kneading) create the protein structures that give dough its plasticity. Once the water is locked up in the amylopectin reservoirs, this lubricant helps keep the dough moist and counteracts some of the stickiness. Health-wise, it's a shade better than Play-Doh's lubricant in the 1960s: deodorized kerosene!

Fragrance
Ah, the childhood memories triggered by that sweet Play-Doh smell. Hasbro's patent admits to vanilla aroma, but that may be just to throw us off the scent. The real formula for this iconic odor is guarded like the crown jewels. After talking with New York perfumer Christopher Brosius, who offers a Play-Doh fragrance, we suspect that it draws from the aromatic flowers of the heliotrope, a.k.a. the cherry pie plant, mixed with the sodium tang of salt and (probably) a combination of acetaldehyde, 2-methylpropanol, and 3-methylbutanol: the gentle aroma of dough itself.

Aluminum Sulfate
In baking, this astringent is used to leaven dough and can act as a stiffener to brace or scaffold the wheat's gluten molecules. Bonus: it imparts a bitter taste, ensuring that hungry or curious preschoolers who take a bite of Play-Doh don't make that mistake twice.

Borax

This alkaline mineral is a common household cleaning—and ant-killing—product. It has antiseptic properties, and Play-Doh's 1965 patent suggests that it's the preferred means of preventing bacteria and mold growth. Though borax is banned in the US as a food additive, Play-Doh is not a food, no matter how much of it you may have eaten over the years. (Borax is also used in Iran to preserve caviar.)

PEG 1500 Monostearate

Along with the mineral or vegetable oil, a 2004 Play-Doh patent suggests that this white waxy solid could be used to reduce the dough's stickiness without letting it slip into sliminess.

Color

When introduced in 1956, Play-Doh came only in dough color. Red, blue, and yellow were added the next year, and a rainbow of other hues followed. Now it's available in forty-three colors, and all of them meet the American Society for Testing and Materials standard for nontoxicity.

[BACKSTORY]

While researching this piece, I learned that Play-Doh is opaque to X-rays. Let's say that again so it sinks in: Play-Doh. Is opaque. To high-energy particles. Like X-rays. It came about like this: A parent ran to the emergency room after their child had swallowed a lump of the stuff. The doctors took an X-ray, and lo and behold there was the lump of Play-Doh, perfectly visible as an opaque splotch in the kid's abdomen. The doctors gathered some more data about Play-Doh and X-rays and immediately wrote a learned paper about their finding.

An X-ray is really pretty simple. Your soft tissues, like skin and organs, are mostly transparent to X-rays, which pass right through them. Hard structures, like bone, are opaque to X-rays and absorb them, which is why bones show up as white on an X-ray. Play-Doh, while soft like flesh, is also an X-ray absorber. Does this mean that if your local nuclear power plant suddenly explodes, you'll be safe if you coat your room in a layer of Play-Doh? Not exactly. It means that if you swallow a lump of Play-Doh that is causing distress, the doctors can put you under the X-ray emitter and actually see the lump of Play-Doh as it makes its way down your gastrointestinal tract. If you are of a more devious mind, wouldn't this mean that you could plant things like illegal drugs, stolen jewelry, or more than three ounces of shampoo inside a lump of Play-Doh to get it past an airport scanner? We're not saying.

But wait a minute. Play-Doh is essentially *dough*. Flour and water. What would make it opaque to X-rays? I personally was of the opinion that it was the borax that did it. Boron is a nuclear moderator, commonly used in reactor control

OSMOSIS

Why does putting salt on a slug kill it? Is salt poisonous to a slug's biochemistry? Not really. Salt kills slugs by the mechanical process of osmosis.

Imagine a system in which the same amount of salt water and freshwater share a common membrane that lets water pass between them but not salt. The freshwater side of the container has more water molecules than the saltwater side, because on the saltwater side, some of the water molecules have been replaced with salt molecules. Since the freshwater side has more water pressure than the saltwater side, some of the water molecules will move across the membrane into the saltwater side, making it fresher than it was. This process is called osmosis, and it stops when the pressure on both sides of the membrane is equal.

Living creatures use osmosis as an easy way to obtain water from the environment. Your kidneys use osmotic pressure to concentrate toxins out of your blood and into urine. Plants use osmosis to take in water: a wet soil environment has a high osmotic pressure, which pushes water into the roots.

And that's what kills the slug. When you sprinkle salt on a slug, the slug's environment immediately changes. Instead of pulling water into the slug's body, osmotic pressure inside the slug now forces water out of the slug's skin, to where the salt is. The salted slug dies not from chemical poisoning but from lack of water.

rods to absorb high-energy subatomic particles. It should have no problem absorbing X-rays.

Unfortunately, despite all my effort, I could never verify the *exact* source of Play-Doh's X-ray opacity: it seems that in all the years this stuff has been on the market, no scientist, as far as I could find, ever had the time and inclination to do the work to break it down and find out the exact reason. And without evidence, there's no story, so we had to leave this information out. However, if you're a qualified nuclear technician with legal access to an X-ray source and some free time on your hands, we'd love to hear from you!

Preparation H

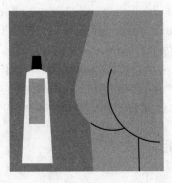

Petrochemical lubricants, nasal decongestant, and the souls (or at least the livers) of dead sharks.

Petrolatum

Folk remedies for hemorrhoids include the application of clarified butter, avoiding cheese, or using jellied soaps on the affected area. Preparation H doesn't use any of these: it uses Vaseline (more precisely, the generic form of the stuff) as a protectant, a mixer, and a delivery medium for the other ingredients. One drawback: petrolatum melts at butt temperature, which can be messy.

Thyme Oil

Elastin is a macromolecule that keeps your body's tissues tight. Inflammation causes white blood cells to produce the enzyme elastase, which breaks down elastin, and with the elastin gone, the affected tissues swell up. Enter thymol, a thyme-oil derivative that blocks elastase production, keeping elastin whole, which keeps certain tissues in your butt from swelling.

Phenylephrine HCl

Applied locally, this vasoconstrictor sends a message to the alpha-adrenergic sites on your neurons to constrict your blood vessels, relax your intestines, and contract all your sphincters. It's also used in nasal decongestants. (We don't recommend Preparation H for a stuffy nose.) This stuff is so powerful that Preparation H now carries a warning label for people like hypertensives and diabetics who may wish to consider whether they should use a drug with all these side effects.

Light Mineral Oil

Hemorrhoids are swollen and inflamed veins in and around the anus. Friction between them and other parts of the body when sitting or walking, as well as periodic contact with, uh, toxic sludge, makes them burn like Catholic guilt. Mineral oil coats the area, reducing friction. It also thins the petrolatum, making the product easier to put on.

Propylparaben

Take benzoic acid, add another -OH group at the bottom and an alkyl group (C_3H_5 in this case) at the top, and you've got a paraben, an inexpensive preservative.

Shark Liver Oil

Harvested from the livers of sharks that live in cold, deep water, this substance is slightly heavier than mineral oil and contains significant quantities of vitamins A and D3, putting it high on the FDA Hemorrhoidal Panel's list of active ingredients for use as protectants in over-the-counter anorectal drug products. Of course, this doesn't begin to touch on the whole moral question of whether or not you should have a deepwater shark killed just to put out the fire in your ass. In the tube, shark liver oil serves as an emulsifier to keep things mixed. In the anal canal, it serves as a barrier against contamination and as a lubricant to cut down on friction and keep things, well, moving along smoothly.

. . . .

Benzoic Acid

A simple six-carbon ring attached to a carboxyl (-COOH) group, benzoic acid penetrates microbial cell membranes, killing any microscopic creature that might feed on Preparation H's biological oils and waxes.

. . . .

Methylparaben

Occurring naturally in blueberries, this antifungal agent degrades easily in UV light, forming oxides that can damage skin, sort of like an antisunscreen. Good thing we use this stuff where the sun doesn't shine.

. . . .

222

[BACKSTORY]

This was easily the most disgusting research I've ever done because, of course, in order for me to understand how hemorrhoids are cured, I had to understand everything there is to know about how they're caused. I'm just made that way. The problem is, I didn't really want to know how hemorrhoids are caused, and I certainly didn't want to know about their complications, and I will only say this—do not do a Google image search of the phrase "pedunculated hemorrhoids" if you have eaten at any time in the past week, because you will surely lose your lunch. This piece was easily far more disgusting than the one about dandruff shampoo.

From its creation in the 1930s, Preparation H had used a special yeast extract to shrink the swelling of hemorrhoidal tissues. It apparently worked well for more than fifty years,

---

ATOMS

Atoms fit into a kind of awkward place, both in nature and in this book. Most of the chemical reactions we talk about in this book do not occur between atoms, but between their constituent parts, like protons, electrons, and neutrons. The peculiar taste of " sour" on your tongue, for instance, comes from an abundance of protons in your saliva interacting with taste bud receptors. On the other end of the scale, many of the larger effects that we talk about in this book take place between molecules, which are self-contained collections of atoms. One atom of nitrogen, for example, combined with three atoms of hydrogen creates a molecule of ammonia, which can interact with a great many other molecules to produce everything from fertilizer to plastic. But none of these effects would be possible without atoms.

but in the early 1990s the FDA stepped in. They claimed that the yeast extract didn't work (more precisely, that there was no evidence that the yeast extract worked as was claimed) and forced the Preparation H company to substitute phenylephrine, which some people consider to be a less effective and slightly more dangerous active ingredient than the yeast extract.

But not every country feels this way. If you are one of the millions of Americans who have your prescription medication shipped to you from Canada to save money, ask the pharmacist to throw in a couple of tubes of their Preparation H; the Canadian version still uses the original formula and doesn't contain any controversial shark liver oil.

Also, I want you to think about this very carefully the next time you are upset about your job. Somewhere in this world there is a man or a woman who sits on the FDA's Hemorrhoidal Panel and serves as their expert in over-the-counter anorectal drug products. You think *your* job blows ass?

This Is What You Put on Your Insects

Lemon Scent Raid

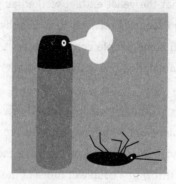

Kills bugs dead with nerve toxin, petroleum, and lemons!

Pyrethrin

This poison causes the ion channels in nerve cells to remain open too long, which makes neurons fire repeatedly, resulting in paralysis and death. Essentially, any bug that absorbs this stuff dies of extreme excitement. It's a pretty vicious outcome, especially when you think of where this chemical comes from: pyrethrin is obtained from the pretty pink-and-white flowers of the asteraceae family (including daisies and chrysanthemums).

Pyrethroids

Pyrethroids are just synthetic pyrethrin. While both are especially toxic to insects (alas, even bees—for a while pyrethroids were believed to be implicated in Colony Collapse Disorder, the increasing disappearance of honeybees since the mid-2000s), they are supposed to be among the least deadly pesticides to mammals. Still, keep Raid away from kitty: cats' livers can't process pyrethrin fast enough to keep them from, you know, dying.

Piperonyl Butoxide or N-octyl Bicycloheptene Dicarboximide

The previous two chemicals, though highly toxic to insects, are pretty easily broken down in an insect's body. This makes any use of the pesticide a race to see if the bug can neutralize the poison before the poison neutralizes the bug. To rig the game, piperonyl butoxide is added to Raid. Not a poison by itself, piperonyl butoxide blocks the action of the insect enzyme that breaks down pyrethrin and pyrethroids. Bugs haven't got a chance.

Isoparaffinic Hydrocarbon Solvent

The patent for Raid recommends Exxsol D60, a proprietary goo concocted by ExxonMobil Chemical and described as an "aliphatic hydrocarbon"—a hydrocarbon without aromatic ring molecules. Here it serves as an oily poison-delivery system that coats the insect's exoskeleton, helping to get the toxins into the pest's pores.

Fragrance

Unscented Raid smells like a kerosene spill in a nerve gas factory. Lemon Scent Raid smells like a kerosene spill in a nerve gas factory, with a hint of lemon.

Sorbitan Monooleate

Older spray pesticides were up to 80 percent hydrocarbons, which aren't the greatest chemicals to be spraying around your house. Raid's current formula cuts the amount of hydrocarbons in half, replacing them with water. Surfactants like sorbitan monooleate help the H_2O and remaining hydrocarbons stay mixed properly.

Sodium Nitrite or Sodium Benzoate

These substances (particularly sodium nitrite) can be toxic in high doses, and in fact they used to be the killing agents in old-fashioned pesticides in the 1940s. But the amounts present here are only enough to prevent the metal can from corroding.

Liquefied Saturated Hydrocarbons

Raid uses a mix of propylene, butanes, and butylenes as propellant. These are flammable and can cause breathing difficulties; you might want to stub out that Marlboro Light before spraying indoors.

ATP

A.k.a. adenosine triphosphate, a.k.a. "life juice." This is the high-energy molecule that powers nearly all of our cellular activities. It is produced in the mitochondria of cells, out of phosphorus, sugars, and fats that the body has taken in as food. ATP is made by at least two distinct processes: in one process, the mitochondria convert one molecule of glucose into 30 molecules of ATP, with carbon dioxide as a waste product. In another process, one molecule of fatty acid is converted to 106 ATP molecules. ATP is then dispersed throughout the cells of the body, where it powers things like basic cellular metabolism, muscle contractions, the creation of DNA, and protein manufacture.

[BACKSTORY]

Imagine you're a Sumerian peasant farmer, about six thousand years ago. Your farm is under siege from insects who believe it is their manifest destiny to eat your crops. You appeal to a local priestess for help. She advises you to try spreading elemental sulfur on your plants.

Or imagine you're an Indian peasant farmer around two thousand years ago. Your crops are also being devoured by insects. You turn to the sacred text of the Rig Veda, book 7, hymn 50, and you learn that praying to all the gods, as well as using "the poison that plants produce," will help in ridding your field of the scorpion and the winding worm.

Almost since the dawn of agriculture, humans have been using pesticides to rid their crops of unwanted pests. Some, like the Greco-Roman practice of burning crabs to cure plant mildew, weren't very effective. Others, like the Chinese trick of spraying arsenic and mercury to control lice, wound up killing more than just the lice. The chemical revolution of the nineteenth century brought new types of pesticides to industrial farms, and, later, into our houses.

This Is What You Put on Your Windshield

Rain-X

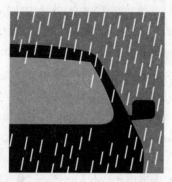

*Rain, rain, go away, polydimethylsiloxane groups
are here to stay. On your windshield.*

Ethanol

That big jug of Rain-X is up to 86 percent sweet biting ethanol.
Since the active ingredients in Rain-X work only if applied to a
clean, dry surface, it's a good thing that all of the ingredients
are dissolved in this alcohol; not only is ethanol a really good
solvent, it helps remove dirt and oil from the glass. Then it
evaporates twice as easily as water would, leaving behind the
active ingredients.

Isopropanol

Rubbing alcohol (though computer geeks know isopropanol as
the smelly solvent for CPU thermal grease). Some poor souls
will try drinking anything to get drunk, so to keep them from
chugging ethanol-rich Rain-X, the company adds this stuff—
it shares a few chemical properties with its cocktail-friendly
cousin, but it's an unpalatable poison. Mixologize with Rain-X
and you'll end up more than just under the weather; more likely
six feet underground.

Polydimethylsiloxane (PDMS)

This substance is a polymer, a chain of repeating molecular subunits. In this case, two organic methyl (CH_3) groups are attached to inorganic silicon-oxygen (SiO). The SiO part forms a thin protective layer on the windshield, while the methyl groups provide low surface tension, which actively repels high-surface-tension fluids like water. These two groups provide a double-strength "*Get lost*" to any raindrops that have the nerve to land on your windshield.

- -

Ethyl Sulfate

While Rain-X is being made in the factory, the scientists add sulfuric acid to the mix (for reasons we'll explain later). By the time the jug reaches your auto parts store, some of the acid has mixed with ethanol and converted to this relatively harmless by-product. It does nothing for Rain-X, since it's just an accidental by-product. One interesting tidbit: it is also found in the urine of alcoholics.

- -

Chlorotrimethylsilane

You've just bought some expensive electronic device. You ceremonially unbox it, and along with the device, out come two packets of something called silica gel. They're included to absorb any excess moisture that might get into the box and ruin the electronic gadget. You know what happens when those water-absorbing silica gel packets actually absorb water? They dissolve into this stuff. A residue from PDMS synthesis, this compound is regularly used to silanize—that is, chemically neutralize—laboratory glassware so that organic molecules won't stick to them. Does it do the same here, for your windshield? A Rain-X chemist told us he couldn't say for sure.

- -

Siloxanes and Silicones, di-Me, Hydroxy-Terminated

When sulfuric acid goes to work on PDMS, it breaks down the long silicon-oxygen-silicon-oxygen chains into smaller segments. The result is this stuff—small fragments of dimethylsiloxane with one very important difference: the chains end with a reactive hydroxyl (-OH) group. These hydroxyl groups help them bond strongly to glass, making it tougher for your wipers to wipe off the Rain-X.

ORGANIC (COMPOUNDS, NOT FOODS)

The old high school chemistry definition is that organic compounds are those substances that contain a carbon atom. However, that doesn't work anymore, because there are plenty of carbon compounds that are *not* considered organic. A more nuanced but unofficial definition says that organic substances contain carbon *and* hydrogen atoms.

Since there is no official definition of "organic," at least in the chemical realm, we'll stick with the nuance: *most* substances that contain carbon (and all that contain a carbon-hydrogen bond) could be considered organic. In the context of chemistry, "organic" doesn't necessarily have anything to do with life: some organic compounds are not found in any living being, and many living creatures contain compounds that would not be considered organic.

A lack of an official definition of "organic" means there isn't one for "inorganic" either. The most common definition of an inorganic compound is "a compound that is not organic"; that is, it does not contain carbon or a carbon-hydrogen bond.

Bob Woodward and Carl Bernstein, the two *Washington Post* reporters who broke the Watergate story in the 1970s, had it easy. Remember how, in *All the President's Men,* they would call up places like the CIA or the Committee for the Re-election of the President and ask to speak to the guy in charge and a few minutes later he would be on the phone? And when they went to visit government workers who may have had some information about Watergate, both the reporters and the sources operated under a commonly accepted understanding of the First Amendment: If a source wanted to talk to a reporter, he or she simply talked to a reporter. If they didn't want to talk, they didn't.

Ask any reporter if those things happen anymore.

The environment for talking to sources has all changed: while the Constitution says that Congress shall make no law infringing the freedom of the press, it says nothing about corporations doing exactly the same thing. And corporations know it: since the 1970s, big companies have come down hard on their employees' relationship with the news media.

An interview request to any sizable organization nowadays consists of talking to the media liaison person first, who then takes four days to set up a speakerphone interview with the person you want to talk to and stays in the room while the interview is going on, causing these weird longish pauses after each question you ask, where you just know they've got their hands over the microphone and are whispering like someone conferring with counsel when testifying before Congress. After the pause they come back and say, "We can't really talk about that, but we'd love to tell you about our new strategic direction . . . ," and as a reporter you sometimes listen to their pitch but mostly you don't, because all you can think about is how you gambled waiting four days for this interview and lost.

Many of you reading this probably already operate under such a stricture: somewhere in your employee orientation handbook, you have been told that you are not allowed to talk to the media about work-related things without first clearing it through your company's media department.

Rain-X is put out by a corporation called SOPUS Products, which used to be Pennzoil–Quaker State but now happens to be a wholly owned subsidiary of Royal Dutch Shell. In a big megacorporation like that, you can usually bet that the "no talking to reporters" rule is strongly enforced. But somewhere out there, there is an unknown chemist who should be proud. He went out on a limb and spoke to this crusading journalist, meeting me like Deep Throat at midnight in abandoned parking lots throughout the Houston area, and at great risk to life and limb he leaked the contents of Rain-X to an unsuspecting world!

Okay, it wasn't that dramatic. In reality, all I did was manage to find an online phone directory for the company. I searched for the most likely department to hold a chemist who worked on Rain-X and I started cold-calling numbers. I think the chemist I spoke to (who shall remain safe behind the pseudonym "Tex," to protect his job) was simply the first one to answer his phone. I said I was a reporter and asked if he knew anything about Rain-X because I needed someone to explain it to me for an article I was writing. He said he sure did; what did I want to know? I said I needed every ingredient explained to me. Tex said he didn't have the ingredient list in front of him. I said I had the list, and I could read off each ingredient if he had the time. He said he sure did.

We spoke on the phone for about forty-five minutes, and Tex was invaluable in helping us understand the complicated process of keeping the rain off your windshield. Our chemist friend either didn't get that memo about not talking to reporters, or he got it and forgot. Or he's just an open, friendly guy who likes his work and likes to talk about it. These days, that alone is enough to make him a rarity.

Unknown chemist, we salute you!

Sta-Green Tree and Shrub Planting Mix

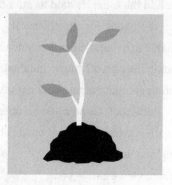

This blessed plot, this earth, this realm, this collection of rotting biosolids.

Reed-Sedge Peat

Good soil is made of rotted organic material. According to the International Peat Society, peat is plant material decaying in an oxygenless, watery bog; this particular type is made of at least 50 percent reeds and sedges (instead of the usual moss). In agriculture, peat is spread over farmland, where it retains water and nutrients to help young plants grow. While still in the bog, peat can remove iron and other heavy metals from polluted water. (Leave it in a bog for a few million years and apply pressure, and it eventually turns into coal.)

Composted Rice Hulls

Rice hulls have almost no nutrients, they don't burn well, and they don't even rot easily. Sure, you can use them as building insulation, or soak the hulls in acid to extract their silica and use that to make solar panels, but that's about the end of their usefulness. Until you compost them. Then they turn into low-pH organic sponges, able to absorb (and slowly release) many times their weight in water—exactly what good garden soil needs to do.

Composted Pine Bark (in Georgia)

Different places around the world have different soil requirements; more to the point, different state and local governments in the US have different prohibitions and permissions regarding what a manufacturer can sell as garden soil. Georgia allows the use of pine bark, which is usually infested with various strains of *Trichoderma,* a fungal double agent working for us in the war against slime. *Trichoderma* produces antibiotics that kill harmful plant fungi in the soil; it also produces enzymes that feed the growing plant's root systems. Pine bark itself creates air spaces in the soil, helping water to reach the roots.

Composted Forest Products (in California)

Did you imagine Black Forest elves bringing their collected bracken to a composting cottage in West Hollywood? Think again. This is mostly lumberyard tailings rotting under anaerobic conditions, much like peat. Why specifically "forest products"? Under EPA guidelines, commercial compost can be made from municipal sewage (the city of Austin, which does this, earned a tidy sum every time you took a dump at South by Southwest).

Potassium Nitrate

Saltpeter, as it's most commonly known, is an ingredient in everything from gunpowder and fireworks to corned beef and desensitizing toothpaste. Its nitrogen and potassium stimulate root growth and activate essential enzymes.

Ammonium Phosphate

A combination of ammonia and phosphoric acid, this provides plants with the P in the chemical ATP, also known as adenosine triphosphate, the chief carrier of energy in living things. Without phosphorus, leaves are stunted and fall off early, roots wither, fewer shoots sprout, and less fruit is produced. Basically, lack of this stuff is like a biblical plague.

Urea

With a name like "urea," you can guess where it comes from, and why farmers let animals pee on their fields. This compound provides a source of nitrogen for mature trees and shrubs, though it may be a little strong for seedlings. Industrially, it's made from ammonia and CO_2. Regardless of the source, in crystalline form it's odorless, colorless, and relatively nontoxic.

Canadian Sphagnum Peat Moss

This is the layer of dead, decomposing sphagnum moss beneath the living layer in the stinky muskeg swamps of the Great White North. Here it acts as a conditioner, aerating compact soils and binding sandy ones, helping each type to hold the optimum amount of air, water, and nutrients that growing plants need.

Ground Dolomitic Limestone

Peat, sphagnum, and various composts in this mix can have a tendency to acidify the soil. This stone—containing calcium magnesium carbonate—buffers soil pH and provides calcium (which promotes strong cell walls) and magnesium (the metal at the heart of the chlorophyll molecule).

Potassium Sulfate

Potassium is a plant macronutrient, along with nitrogen and phosphorus. Without it, the complex multistep process of photosynthesis doesn't work efficiently, particularly when water is scarce. Plants use sulfur to activate enzymes, as well as to manufacture cysteine and methionine, two amino acids important for producing protein.

[BACKSTORY]

This piece started with the expectation that dirt was dirt was dirt. Really, how many different ingredients can there be in a bag of dirt? Before I knew it, I was making multiple trips to the Science, Industry and Business branch of the New York Public Library on Madison Avenue in Manhattan, as well as initiating phone calls and e-mails with chemists, agricultural experts, marketing experts, and government officials from the state of Florida (to whom I sent an e-mail with the subject line "Media inquiry about cow manure"—it is a liberating thing for the soul to be able to send a government official an e-mail with a subject line about cow manure).

PHOTOSYNTHESIS

This is the source of all food on Earth. A surprisingly complicated process, photosynthesis takes place in chloroplasts, small specialized subunits of plant cells. These bodies contain chlorophyll, the active biomolecule of photosynthesis. Chlorophyll most easily absorbs photons of light in the blue part of the spectrum, specifically the exact wavelength of a bright blue sky. Plants do not necessarily absorb sunlight as much as they absorb *skylight*. Chlorophyll also absorbs some red light and reflects green light (which is why plants look green). These photons power the entire photosynthesis system, which also requires carbon dioxide and water. The chloroplasts recombine these three inputs into carbohydrates, water, and leftover oxygen. Sometimes the carbohydrates are stored in the plant's sweet, juicy fruits; sometimes they are recombined to make things like cellulose (as in cotton or linen) or wood. Depending on the species of plant, the water can be stored, as in cacti, or released to the atmosphere. The oxygen produced by photosynthesis is released into the atmosphere.

Whatever happened to dirt was dirt was dirt? As it turns out, you can make soil out of almost anything that can be composted.

That includes things like human waste. It is perfectly legal to compost and sell human waste as a garden product. The process is very carefully regulated by the EPA, and the resulting stuff even has its own name: biosolids. As mentioned in the story, the city of Austin, Texas, really has been sterilizing, composting, bagging, and selling its own biosolids since 1989.

I want to make it very clear that this product does not use composted human waste; none of the garden soils I looked at did, at least not in a way that was clearly defined on the label. I was told off the record by an industry official that they unequivocally do not and will not ever use sewage compost for just that reason—they're afraid people won't buy human shit, and they're even more afraid of the backlash if they use a term like "biosolids" and people later discover that they've been filling their garden in human feces all along. Besides, how can you come up with the right advertising campaign to sell Americans their own poop back to them?

Tide Pods

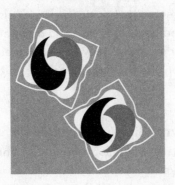

Glue bubbles, voracious enzymes, and a dazzling fluorescent dye.

Polyvinyl Alcohol

This is the "pod" itself, a plasticlike membrane that holds the other ingredients in a jolly candylike form. (Reportedly, it's so candylike that hundreds of kids have attempted to eat these and wound up with a gob full of detergent.) It's a water-soluble polymer similar to Elmer's Glue: pop it in the wash and it dissolves, releasing detergenty goodness without any messy spills. Tide says its three-chambered design "maximizes the consumer experience," which probably means keeping the ingredients separated so that they don't neutralize each other while sitting on the shelf.

Fatty Acid Salts

A.k.a. soap, because corporate America won't use one syllable when it can use five. It works by attaching its hydrocarbon chains to the grease or oil in a clothing stain, allowing both to be washed away by water.

Alcoholethoxy Sulfate

Any one of several linear anionic surface-acting agents (which the laundry industry calls "surfactants," which is just a fancy name for "detergents") that doing the laundry is all about. As with soap, one end binds to grease and dirt that's stuck to your clothes; the other end binds to water molecules in the washing machine. Agitation lifts the stain off the fabric, to be banished down the drain.

Disodium Distyryl-Biphenyl Disulfonate

This substance makes your clothes brighter! And whiter! Actually, all it makes is an optical illusion. DDD absorbs ultraviolet light with a wavelength in the range 340–360 nanometers (known as UV-A, the really bad ultraviolet). It then takes its absorbed energy and fluoresces (i.e., emits light) at around 440–460 nanometers, giving your clothes a faint blue glow. This blueness counteracts the natural yellowing of old clothes, to make them look whiter and brighter. There's just one drawback: US soldiers had to be specifically instructed to wash their fatigues in a DDD-free detergent, since its glow was making their uniforms show up when viewed through night-vision goggles.

Mannanase

The specific class of enzymes used in detergents are the Terminators of the laundry world, relentlessly catalyzing whatever substances they're aimed at. This enzyme can break apart guar gum, a thickener used in ice cream and salad dressing—and in fluids for hydraulic fracking—which can leave behind hard-to-remove stains.

Termamyl and Natalase

Two types of amylase, which are enzymes that break apart starch-based stains like those from gravy and baby food.

Termamyl is the high-temperature variant, natalase the low. Together they get the job done in hot, warm, and cold water.

Xyloglucanase

This enzyme breaks down the cellulose in plant cell walls. It also slows the formation of little pills or fuzz on natural-fiber materials like cotton or linen. The idea is that this enzyme chews up the fine, tendril-like fibers sticking out of the clothing (a process Tide calls "polishing" the fabric).

Subtilisin

Face it—some clothing stains come directly from your filthy human body. This enzyme (an excretion of *Bacillus subtilis* or *Bacillus licheniformis*) breaks down stains caused by left-behind keratin found mostly in the dead outer layer of skin cells, which contributes to the grime a previous generation knew as ring around the collar.

Diethylene Triamine Pentaacetate Sodium

This is a chelant—a molecule that latches on to metals. (The last time you went to the hospital for a nuclear scan, you probably were injected with this stuff, which keeps the radioactive particles from sticking around in your body when the test is over.) If your wash water is hard, this softens it, enabling the enzymes and surfactants to work more effectively. It also lifts stains that contain metal ions—like blueberries—and keeps them from re-adhering to your duds.

Calcium Formate

Enzymes are voracious beasts; on their own, their need for destruction is so great they will even devour themselves over time. They can also become inactive when exposed to heat. To help ensure they're still around when you need them, this substance is added to keep the enzymes "folded" until the pod is used. In the wash, it just floats away, leaving the enzymes free to assault your bespattered clothing.

. . . .

Polyethyleneimine Ethoxylate

Just think of it as a chelant for nonmetals; this polymer (and other polymers in the ingredient list) works with the surfactants to break up soil that comes off your clothes. Polymers then wrap themselves around the dirt, preventing it from redepositing onto your clothes and making sure it all comes out in the wash.

. . . .

DETERGENTS

One hundred years ago, World War I was tearing apart the great nations of Europe. Nearly all the basics of life were in short supply. Plant and animal fats were badly needed for the war effort; their natural glycerins could be used to make nitroglycerin explosives. But soap is made out of fats, and the resulting lack of soap in the shops horrified the normally fastidious German people. They put their chemists to work inventing a soap substitute that doesn't need fats. The chemists responded by combining propyl or butyl alcohols with naphthalene and then adding sulfur to make a detergent that was . . . not very good. Continued research in the 1920s and 1930s with other chemicals resulted in the first workable nonsoap shampoos and detergents, just in time for World War II. Artificial detergents for household use really took off in the postwar years with the development of the first synthetic laundry detergent, Tide.

[BACKSTORY]

I t used to be a common-enough trope in movies and TV shows: if you screw up enough times in the military, as punishment they assign you to the public affairs office. I have no idea if that is still the case, but it was a very unhappy-sounding officer who answered the phone at the US Army's Media Relations Division. I said I was calling to see if soldiers had any restrictions about the detergent they could use to wash their uniforms.

I was calling at the tail end of the US military's active combat presence in Iraq. The press office was probably being bombarded by media questions about combat deaths, combat injuries, the status of deployments, and the like. And then suddenly in comes this off-the-wall question about . . . "Let me understand this," the officer shouted, "you're seriously asking me if they are allowed to do their laundry in . . . in *Tide*?"

"Yes, sir," I said. "That is exactly what I asked."

I had a mental image of his seething inside, asking heaven, "Why do I have to deal with this Mickey Mouse shit!?!?" We went back and forth—him demanding more information as to just *why* I was so curious about soldiers' uniforms, me wondering why he was so agitated—until he eventually shouted that he'd have to get back to me with that information.

I'm still waiting.

The rest of the piece was pretty fun. Once again I had to deal with Procter & Gamble, this time in their role as the makers of Tide. For some of the previous articles I've done, I would categorize P & G's attitude as less than helpful. For this one, however, they did a complete turnaround: they hooked me up with three scientists and a PR person, and as far as I could tell, the scientists had no restrictions about which of my questions they could answer. Of course, for each scientific answer I got from the scientists, the PR lady kept saying things like, "We leveraged our surfactant models to provide consumers with a Tide experience that meets or surpasses their aesthetic as well as their cleansing expectations," twenty-four words with basically no meaning. But the really interesting thing is that this turnaround in P & G's attitude toward my questions came at about the same time they started to list all the ingredients for all their products on their website. Were my columns a part of that?

Titleist Golf Balls

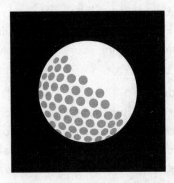

Dense, flexible, and resilient. As balls should be.

Cis-1,4-Polybutadiene

It's rubber with a memory. This polymer's chain of repeating units are cis-linked—that is, they are all connected on the same side of a carbon-carbon double bond. Once molded into a shape (like a ball), the material returns to that shape whenever it gets deformed (like when it's hit by a golf club). This provides outstanding resiliency—modern golf balls spring back into shape in just a thousandth of a second.

Trans-Polyisoprene

Grandpa called this stuff gutta-percha, a form of hard rubber from Southeast Asian trees. A polymer of isoprene (natural latex rubber), TPI is different from most rubbers in that the isoprene units are trans-linked (connected on opposite sides of the carbon-carbon link). That makes it stiffer than normal cis-polyisoprene, perfect for things that shouldn't deform. TPI revolutionized golf when "gutties" appeared in 1848; these hard rubber balls were cheaper, easier to make, and more durable than what duffers used previously: leather balls filled with compressed goose feathers.

Zinc Acrylate

Talk about your one-trick ponies: up to fifty million pounds of this chemical are made in the US every year, and as much as 90 percent of it goes into golf balls. Normal rubber flows under stress and heat, but zinc acrylate forms links across the polybutadiene chains, keeping your balls flexible but solid.

Benzoyl Peroxide

If you had zits any time after the 1970s, you probably remember this stuff as the greatest topical acne medication ever, mowing down bacteria and drying (even peeling!) your skin like nothing else on the market. What's it doing here? It shears electrons from the zinc acrylate and polybutadiene molecules so they can form strong cross-links.

Zinc Oxide

This is the white stuff on a lifeguard's nose. In weak concentrations, as little as 0.5 percent, it can assist the rubber cross-linking process mentioned above. In much stronger concentrations, up to 50 percent, it can serve as a filler, probably to bring the ball as close as possible to the maximum allowed USGA weight of 1.62 ounces without going over. Why this preoccupation with mass? In golf, heavy balls are not a handicap.

Masterbatch Red (or other colors)

Dickens character? Nineties Celtic trip-hop group? Neither. Masterbatches are additives used to impart particular qualities to plastics. There are some that glow in the dark, others that biodegrade, and even a version that repels rats. Here? Nothing more than an easily adjusted filler to keep the mass of the balls just right.

Polyurethane

Finally, all that springy rubber is encased in a sleek, aerodynamic shell of polyurethane elastomer. Used in various formulations in everything from roller skate wheels to drive belts, it combines flexibility with tremendous resistance to abrasion—just what you want in something you're going to beat with a club. This is also where the dimples go—anywhere from 252 to 482 indentations that increase lift and reduce drag on the ball. Just like a spandex swimsuit!

- -

SOLID

A solid consists of a group of molecules held together by strong intermolecular bonds, like an Eastern European ethnic clan. This differs from a gas, in which the molecules are flighty and insincere and not generally held together, or a liquid, in which the bonds holding the molecules together are simpering weak things that allow the liquid to be molded by the situation it finds itself in. Solids are structurally rigid, and they resist deformation when stress is applied; solids do not flow, and they can maintain their own shape, irrespective of any container.

This Is What You Put on Your Baby's Bottom

Triple Paste Diaper Cream

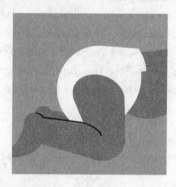

Like waterproofing your basement, except it's your offspring.

Zinc Oxide

ZnO is one of those amazing ingredients that can be used to make everything from paint to dental fillings to sunscreen to spacecraft components. A dirty diaper contains your precious little angel's toxic waste, and zinc oxide—yes, it's the actual mineral zinc—provides a powerful barrier between scum and bum.

Cornstarch

When you marinate in your own urine, as babies do, you have to expect your skin to get waterlogged and pruny. This increase in skin folding leads to an increase in skin friction, which leads to redness and inflammation—leading to the technical term for diaper rash: diaper dermatitis. Cornstarch, if applied directly to the skin, can help absorb some of that liquid, help to reduce the pruning, and therefore help to reduce the rash.

White Petrolatum

This actually comes out of the ground, a waxy black gunk that coats the surface of oil-well drill bits. When it is filtered, it becomes a colorless, odorless, jellylike mass you probably know better by its brand name: Vaseline. Liquids increase the permeability of skin (allowing irritants like urine and fecal enzymes into the epidermis—ouch!), so keeping baby's skin dry, yet not dried out, with a protective coating of this stuff is one key to combating diaper rash.

Anhydrous Lanolin

Brought to you by special glands on a sheep, which exude this stinky yellow oil into their wool as a waterproofing agent (waterproofing, as you've seen, is a recurring theme in diaper rash remedies). It can be purified into lanolin, a wax with a melting point around human body temperature. When applied to a baby's skin, it can also thicken the inner skin layer by accelerating the growth of new cells—exactly what you'd want if you'd been soaking in ammoniated piss all night.

Stearyl Alcohol

Now easily extracted from plants, this eighteen-carbon fatty alcohol used to be distilled from sperm-whale oil. Check your local reservoir—water utilities sometimes float a thin layer of stearyl alcohol on the surface of their reservoirs to retard evaporation. Note the water-barrier theme yet again?

Bisabolol

Granny's folk remedy for diaper rash was to soak the baby's bottom in cool chamomile tea. This compound, extracted from chamomile, penetrates the skin and has anti-inflammatory, antibacterial, and muscle-relaxant properties. The old lady knew what she was talking about.

Oat Kernel Extract

Of all the indignities caused by sitting in your own poop, the worst may be a *Candida* yeast infection (about one-third of children have fecal *Candida*). Many topical antifungal agents may be too harsh for a newborn's skin, but extract of *Avena sativa* seeds contains a very mild antifungal protein that's just right.

. . . .

Cholesterol

This vital component of our cell membranes is the ur-steroid, the material from which progesterone, testosterone, and other hormones are derived. But while some skin creams are steroid based, raw cholesterol has no steroidal power; it is most likely just a moisturizer and emulsifier for keeping all the other ingredients properly mixed.

. . . .

Polysorbate 80

A food additive from the atomic age, when artificial meant better, this chemical has been touted as a baldness cure (unproven), denigrated as a carcinogen (not), and held up as evidence that the flu vaccine is part of a vast government conspiracy (isn't). It's actually just an emulsifier.

. . . .

AMINE

Start with ammonia (NH_3), and knock off at least one of the hydrogen atoms. The remaining substance is an amine—the building block for things like amino acids. In the gaseous phase they smell like ammonia; liquid amines smell kind of fishy (the dead-fish smell is specifically trimethylamine). The human body uses amines to make neurotransmitters like dopamine and serotonin. Chemists use amines to make dyes, plastics, and drugs that act very much like dopamine and serotonin.

[BACKSTORY]

I wrote to the president of the Triple Paste diaper rash cream company to set up an interview to talk about some of the ingredients. I sent him a few sample questions so he would have some idea what we were going to talk about (I'm really not into gotcha journalism unless I catch someone in a lie).

At around this time, the "What's Inside" series was getting to be pretty well-known. It was on a weekly TV show and had been referenced in other print media. Scientists I contacted for information were starting to have heard of it. And corporation people were getting wary—more than one PR person had turned me down when I said the words "What's Inside." I can only assume that that is the reason the president of the Triple Paste company wrote back very politely saying that he thought my questions were excellent, he was sure I would write a wonderful article, and he would not help in any way whatsoever.

You have to respect that.

You also have to respect that new parents are effectively insane about their babies. They want the best for their children, and they want to keep their children safe. Unfortunately, modern product labeling doesn't always help them.

ACKNOWLEDGMENTS

The pieces in this book wouldn't have existed without the editors at *Wired* magazine: starting with Paul Boutin, who got me in the door, and Laura Moorhead, to whom I first pitched the idea of analyzing the ingredient list of everyday products. "What's Inside" itself was edited by the long-suffering Adam Rogers, the long-suffering Rob Capps, the slightly-suffering Nancy Miller, the occasionally-suffering Caitlin Roper, the extraordinarily-long-suffering Chris Baker, and the medium-suffering Jon Eilenberg. These stories were kept going by the unfailing support of Chris Anderson, at the time the editor in chief of *Wired*; and Jacob Young.

Any writer who doesn't love and respect his fact checkers is a fool. Each of these chapters is incredibly information-dense: a six-hundred-word investigation of a product can have as many as sixty or seventy footnotes, all of which need to be independently verified (a "normal" six-hundred-word magazine story will have six, maybe seven footnotes). The fact checkers I've worked with—Erin Biba, Jordan Crucchiola, Erik Malinowski, Jaclyn Mellini, Rachel Swaby, Angela Watercutter, Jenna Wortham, and especially Timothy Lesle, all ruled at the time by the benevolent research editor Joanna Pearlstein—have saved my ass countless times. It comes as no surprise that they all have gone on to become journalism stars in their own right. Yet another reason not to disrespect your fact checkers: you may be working for them some day. Despite their best efforts, any mistakes that remain in this book are mine and mine alone.

Other *Wired* folks, such as Brendan Koerner, Mat Honan, Mark McCluskey, TV's Chris Hardwick, and Noah Schactman (currently of the Daily Beast), were also invaluable in their support.

My agents, Daniel Greenberg and Tim Wojcik at Levine Greenberg Rostan Literary Agency, saw what no other agents saw in a few pages of text and some magazine clippings, and they shepherded me through the wildest four weeks of my life as this book got pitched. Also thanks to business manager Melissa Rowland, and foreign agent (is that the same as spy?) Beth Fisher.

These stories would just be pieces of paper floating in the wind were it not for the patience and enthusiasm of my editor at Three Rivers Press, senior editor Amanda Patten, who shaped these ramblings into a book. Thanks also to Lisa Buch and Jenni Zellner, who held down the fort when Amanda was away. Anders Wenngren's playful and smart illustrations gave the book a dynamism that simple text couldn't achieve. Elizabeth Rendfleisch, who heads the Three Rivers design group, and Cathy Hennessy, the production editor on the book, actually made these words into a real object you can hold in your hands.

A book like this needs lots and lots of input from the public. Some friends and strangers who gave ideas and support are Nancy Krull Aronson, Delva Comizio Assante, Eliene Augenbraun, Peter Barossi, Angela Barranco, Carmen Perez Barton, Lynn Beighley, Stewart Brand, John Brooks, Jean Curtin Brosnan, Tiffany Lee Brown, Lily Burana, Margaret Burke, Jamais Cascio, Michael DeChiara, Salvatore Denaro, Tritia Denaro, Cory Doctorow, Elaine Drebot-Hutchins, Gideon Evans, Lee Felsenstein, Sharon Fisher, Fawn Fitter, Elisa Flynn, James Forde, Mark Frauenfelder, Lucy Gertz, Paul Gertz, Cynthia Heimel, Joe Hobaica, John Hodgman, Robert Howe, Marjorie Ingall, Richard Kadrey, Lisa Volpicelli Kalfus, Amy L. Keyishian, Stephen King, Megan Kingery, Margaret Kranyak, Brian Lam, Jenny Herdman Lando, Eleanor Lang, Beth Zulli Lusuriello, Sarah Lusuriello, Toni

McCloskey, Jeffrey McIntyre, Carrie McLaren, Kristin MacLaughlin, Dan Maskara, Racheline Maltese, Sarah Maybaum, Frances Mercanti-Anthony, Barbara Moroch, Felicity O'Meara, Scott Owens, Linda Pohorence-Walsh, Colette Post, Maura Kenney Rast, Christine Roberson, Douglas Rushkoff, Susan Scott, Gary Shteyngart, Molly Wright Steenson, Alex Steffen, Neil deGrasse Tyson, Mary Wallace, Wil Wheaton, Kevin Wilkinson, Mary Elizabeth Williams, Tom Wolfe, and Carrie Zaitz.

Thanks also to the CEOs, scientists, engineers, professors, and others who willingly sat for an interview or otherwise provided information vital to the cause: Ibrahim Abbas, Dr. Phillip C. Bennet, Lynn Bohan, Mark Boston, Christopher Brosius, Alton Brown, Keri Butler, John Carter, Shellie Porter Caudill, Frank Clark, Anne Coiley, Dr. Joe Cordray, David deFoe, Dr. David J. Hanson, Rob Hardy, Tyler Jeffrey, Jim Koch, Julia Kostecka, Megan Lustig, Geri Lykins, Dr. Harold McGee, Drew McGowan, Stephanie McGuane, Dr. Suzette Middleton, Dr. Sidney Mirvish, Dr. Roshini Rajapaksa, Eric Soderstrom, Ruth Winter, and Mary Woods.

I currently have in my wallet active library cards for the New York Public Library, the Yonkers Public Library, the New York Academy of Medicine Library, the Brooklyn Public Library, as well as a reader identification card issued by the Library of Congress. The research staffs of these and other libraries, as well as the entire Interlibrary Loan (ILL) system, are national treasures.

My sister Melissa Perdock and my brother Andy Di Justo (the real hypochondriac of the family), would let me know when I had hit a nerve by calling me after they had read a breakdown of their favorite snack and screaming "GREAT! Now you've ruined another product for me!"

And as always, extra special thanks and love to Emily Gertz, who made it all feel so easy.